Advanced Geriatric Medicine 7

Edited by

J. Grimley Evans MD DM FRCP FFCM
Professor of Geriatric Medicine, University of Oxford

and

F. I. Caird DM FRCP
David Cargill Professor of Geriatric Medicine,
University of Glasgow

Wright
London Boston Singapore Sydney Toronto Wellington

First published, 1988

© Butterworth & Co. (Publishers) Ltd, 1988

British Library Cataloging in Publication Data

Advanced geriatric medicine.
7
1. Geriatrics
I. Caird, F. I. (Francis Irvine)
II. Evans, J. Grimley (John Grimley)
618.97

ISBN 0-7236-1343-5

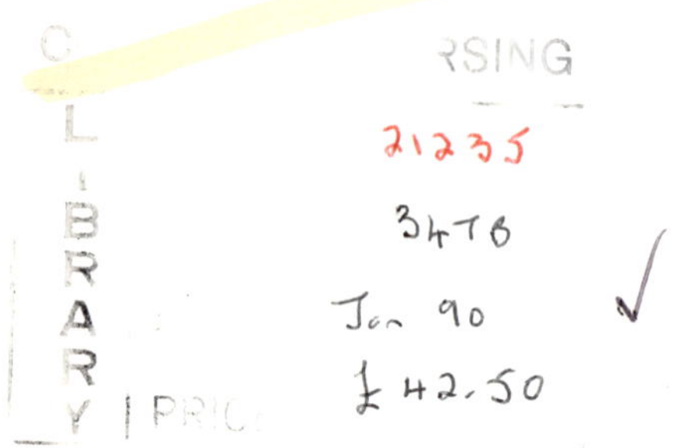

Photoset by Butterworths Litho Preparation Department
Printed and bound in England by Hartnolls Ltd, Bodmin, Cornwall

Preface

The chapters in this volume are based on presentations given in the Advanced Geriatric Medicine Course held in Oxford in the autumn of 1987. One of the themes explored was the applicability of so-called 'high technology medicine' – an infelicitous term – in the care of older people. The needs of elderly people in our society have too long been identified exclusively with prosthetic services and long-term dependency. Elderly people have the right to expect benefit from the technological advances of medicine which they have helped to finance through their working years. This is not to imply that high technology interventions should be applied to elderly people without careful thought (nor, we may hope, to people of any age), but rather that there should not be an equally thoughtless exclusion of elderly people from consideration for therapeutic rather than prosthetic interventions. The need to make our approach to the increasing numbers of elderly patients both more rational and more humane is one of the most serious challenges to medicine in the next decade.

While several of the contributions bear on this issue, we have also included in this volume topics concerned with clinical problems in later life and age-associated changes in physiology. The final contribution brings the study of ageing into the heartland of contemporary medicine by addressing the question of the molecular basis of intrinsic ageing. Geriatric medicine has indeed come a long way from the workhouses of 40 years ago.

J. Grimley Evans
F. I. Caird

Contributors

A. H. Al-Hillawi MD MRCP
Consultant Physician, Stoke Mandeville Hospital

R. N. Barton BSc PhD
Scientist, North West Injury Research Centre, Manchester

M. K. Benson MD FRCP
Consultant Physician, Oxford

J. M. Bone BSc MB FRCP
Consultant Physician, Royal Liverpool Hospital

C. M. Castleden MD FRCP
Professor of Geriatric Medicine, University of Leicester

Keren N. Davies MB MRCP
Registrar in Geriatric Medicine, Leicester General Hospital, Leicester

D. S. Fairweather PhD MRCP
University Lecturer in Geriatric Medicine and Consultant Physician,
Fellow of Corpus Christi College, Oxford

M. Hardman BSc MRCP
Clinical Lecturer in Clinical Pharmacology, University of Oxford

J. R. Hodges MB MRCP
Clinical Lecturer in Neurology, University of Oxford

M. A. Horan PhD MRCP
Senior Lecturer in Geriatric Medicine, University of Manchester

I. G. Kelly BSc MD FRCS
Senior Lecturer in Orthopaedic Surgery, University of Glasgow

R. A. Little BSc PhD MRCPath
Scientific Director, North West Injury Research Centre, Manchester

Michael Lye MD FRCP
Professor of Geriatric Medicine, University of Liverpool

J. B. McDonald MB MRCP
Consultant Physician in Geriatric Medicine, Gartnavel General Hospital, Glasgow

O. J. M. Ormerod DM MRCP
Clinical Lecturer in Cardiology, University of Oxford

J. R. Playfer MD FRCP
Consultant Geriatrician, Royal Liverpool Hospital

R. C. Tallis BM FRCP
Professor of Geriatric Medicine, University of Manchester

S. Westaby BSc MS FRCS
Consultant Cardiothoracic Surgeon, Oxford

Contents

Chapter 1

Pulmonary function tests and ageing

A. H. Al-Hillawi

The aims – and limitations – of this review are to describe those changes in lung function that typically occur with ageing. To do this, it is necessary to have some idea of the concepts underlying these physiological tests and to have some convenient method of expressing their results.

A simple approach is to suppose that the healthy lung is a 'black box' that processes air and venous blood to produce arterial blood of acceptable quality regardless of the quantity or quality of the venous blood presented to it. This concept is based on repeated observations that in nearly all healthy younger adults, even when

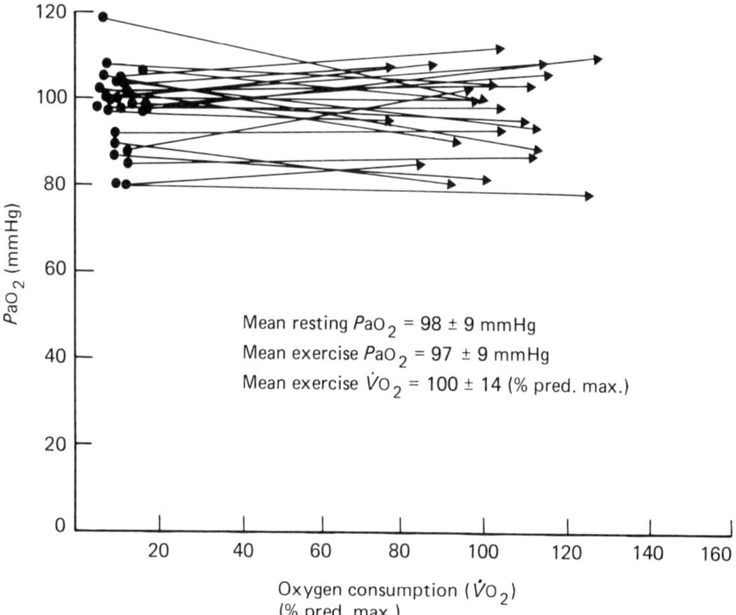

Figure 1.1 Plot of arterial oxygen tension against oxygen consumption in 25 healthy men (mean age 43, s.d. 12 years)

they are exercising maximally, the lungs succeed in producing arterial blood with oxygen and carbon dioxide tensions close to 100 mmHg (13.3 kPa) and 40 mmHg (5.3 kPa), respectively (Figures 1.1, 1.2). The ageing process does not spare the respiratory system, however, and this process may alter the efficiency of our 'black box'. To explain why this should be so, it is helpful to know how the functional state of the lungs is normally described.

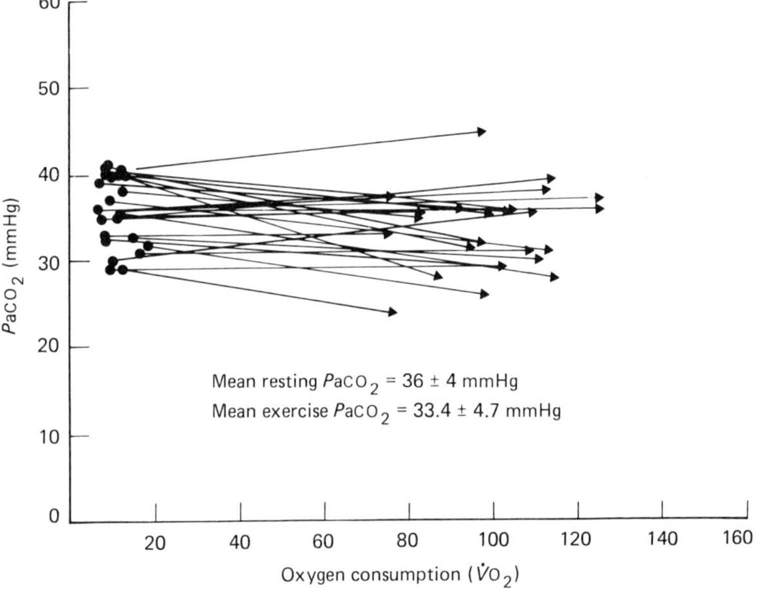

Figure 1.2 Plot of arterial carbon dioxide tension against oxygen consumption in 25 healthy men (mean age 43, s.d. 12 years)

Resting lung function

A healthy person who first inhales completely, exhales as fast and deeply as possible and then inhales completely again as fast as possible, follows the reproducible course of the maximal flow-volume loop (Figure 1.3). Thus there is a rapid rise to peak expiratory flow (PEF) and then a linear fall off of flow until residual volume (RV) is reached. In normal persons PEF occurs in the first tenth of the course from total lung capacity (TLC) to RV and is equal to twice the predicted forced vital capacity (FVC) per second. The volume expired in the first secton (FEV_1) equals 65% to 85% of the FVC. After reaching RV, the loop follows a smooth curve as the subject inhales back to TLC. Peak inspiratory flow (PIF) occurs at mid-inspiration and equals about 1.5 times the predicted FVC/s. If intrathoracic pressures are recorded at the same time, they remain fairly constant throughout expiration indicating that the fall in expiratory flow rate with diminishing lung volume occurs despite strongly maintained expiratory pressure. This fall-off is generally attributed to two factors: progressive airway narrowing and progressive loss of lung recoil.

If TLC is measured by whole-body plethysmography (which senses the compressible gas volume of the lung), the flow-volume loop can be charted on a predicted TLC scale. During plethysmography it is possible to measure mean alveolar gas pressure and respired flow simultaneously and non-invasively. These measurements allow the determination of airway conductance per litre of lung volume (SGAW = flow per litre of driving pressure). Because airway geometry varies widely through the respiratory cycle and is more stable in inspiration, it is usual to measure conductance during the first half-litre of normal inspiration. To match it to the flow-volume loop in Figure 1.3, it is shown by a descending bar on the right of the figure, which should be as deep as the inspiratory limb of the normal loop. Finally, if the subject breathes out to residual volume, then inhales a vital capacity of air containing helium and holds his breath for 10 s at total lung capacity, the helium-marked air travels through the residual volume reaching all but the most distant third in 10 s. The unreached part represents the inaccessible or effectively trapped gas volume. In the absence of low airway conductance (a large-airway characteristic), the inaccessible gas volume becomes a measure of small-airway function. The volume of gas reached by the marked air or accessible gas volume (VA) is shown by the upper horizontal bar in Figure 1.3. Moreover, if the inhaled air is also labelled with low concentrations of carbon monoxide (CO), the uptake of gas can be compared with the almost insoluble helium. The helium measurements allow calculation of the initial partial pressure of CO in the alveoli (PAco) and the final CO concentration after 10 s, measured by sampling late in rapid expiration. From these the transfer factor for carbon monoxide (TLCO), or the rate of transfer of CO per mmHg PAco, is calculable; this is also expressed as CO transfer per litre of accessible gas volume, i.e. TLCO/VA, known as KCO. The TLCO is thought to represent the volume of haemoglobin accessible to the alveolar air[1] or the blood that can be reached by

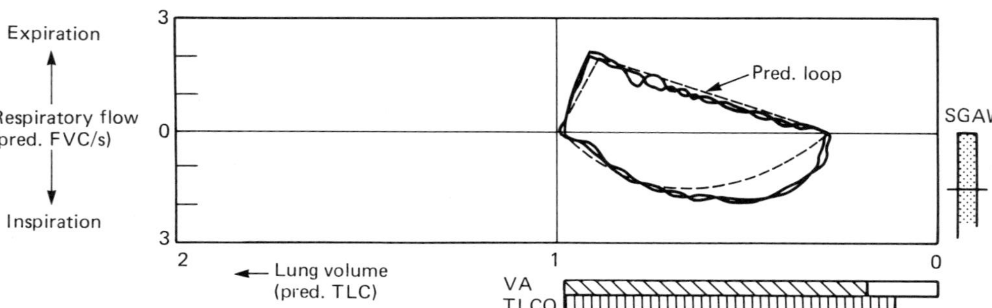

Figure 1.3 Functional characteristics of the lungs of a 30-year-old healthy man

diffusion and is a measure of pulmonary 'very small vessel' blood volume; it is depicted by the lower horizontal bar.

The lungs are dependent on elastin and collagen for their emptying and filling. The lungs have an elaborate network of elastic fibres that run from their effective 'centre' at the base of the larynx along the airways, spreading over each alveolus and eventually terminating in the visceral pleura. This elastic sheath allows for orderly retraction after each inspiration and is therefore important in lung emptying. In contrast, the limit to lung filling is set by collagen fibres lying parallel to the elastic fibres. These collagen fibres are wrinkled throughout most of their volume range, only tautening to their elastic limit as total lung capacity is reached.

Ageing effects

This section describes those changes characteristic of ageing that may be detected by routine lung function tests. Factors other than intrinsic ageing may have an important influence. Cigarette smoking, for example, leaves easily detectable abnormalities in these tests in spite of the smoker's remaining asymptomatic. Figure 1.4 shows the characteristics of 165 healthy men and

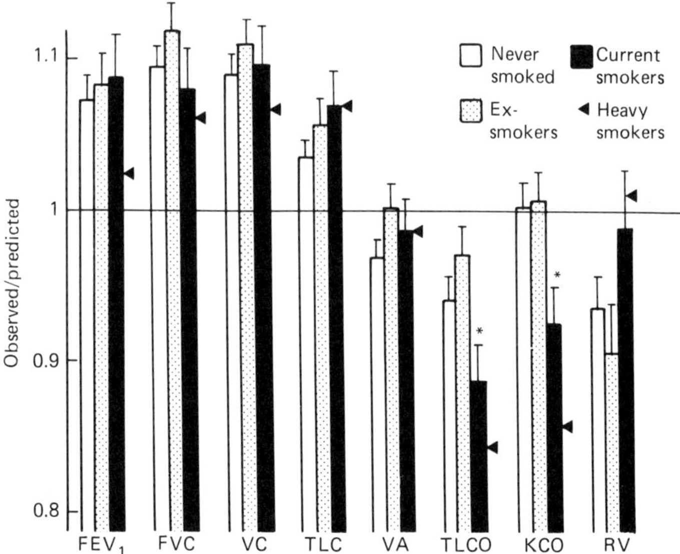

Figure 1.4 Bar chart of lung function (observed/predicted) in 165 healthy men and women identified for smoking habit (heavy smokers are defined as those smoking more than 20 cigarettes per day)

women aged 31 to 60 whose smoking habits had been identified[2]. Heavy smokers (more than 20 cigarettes a day) are seen to have depressed CO transfer and minor increases in TLC and RV, the latter probably due to early small-airways disease causing gas trapping.

Changes in the maximal flow-volume loop

The maximal expiratory flow-volume curve shows an increase in convexity towards the volume axis at low lung volumes relative to younger adults.[3] This change in shape is only evident in the last 30% of the expired VC (Figure 1.5). This is thought to be due to loss of lung recoil with age and is accompanied by an increased resistance to flow in peripheral airways. The recoil forces themselves are important in generating the negative pressures necessary to hold these airways open. It appears that qualitative changes in the structure of collagen fibrils and in elastin may be responsible for the age-associated reduction in elastic recoil of the lung; quantitative alterations in these constituents still have undefined significance in relation to lung physiology[4]. Furthermore, a reduction in surface tension forces, known to occur with increasing age, will decrease elastic recoil and is probably consequent upon a fall in alveolar surface area. As with all skeletal muscle, the strength of respiratory muscles diminishes with age and this too may contribute to lower recoil pressure.

Since healthy adults are able to expire more than 70% of their FVC in the first second, the FEV_1 will include part of those

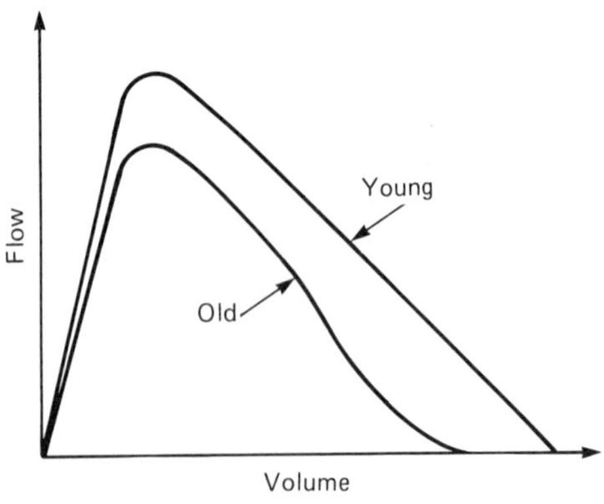

Figure 1.5 Effects of age on the maximal expiratory flow-volume curve

terminal portions of the expiratory flow-volume curve. Thus, the FEV_1 declines with age and the literature suggests that this will occur in a linear fashion by about 30 ml per year in non-smoking men[5] and by 21 ml in non-smoking women. These data largely originate from cross-sectional studies, however, and more recent longitudinal estimates suggest that this fall does not commence until 40 years of age, does not exceed 20 ml until the age of 60 in either sex, and only exceeds 30 ml after the age of 70 in men[6]. In women the latter fall is less marked and may be related to the difference in height between the two sexes. Men tend to be taller and since FEV_1 is proportional to height, the taller person with the larger FEV_1 demonstrates a more rapid decline than a shorter subject.

The peak expiratory flow rate also declines with age, probably by 75–100 l/min between the ages of 30 and 65[7]. It is reached, as noted above, in the first tenth of the journey from TLC to RV and is dependent on muscular pressure and so on effort. At lower volumes, maximum expiratory flow becomes less dependent on the driving pressure. Ageing respiratory muscles are weaker than their younger counterparts and this contributes to lower peak flow.

Lung volumes

The FVC declines with age and the loss per year of age is up to 30 ml in men and 25 ml in women after the fourth decade. Total lung capacity is largely unaffected and since this stays stable while FVC falls, the RV (or 'minimum' lung volume) must rise. The accessible lung volume (VA) is slightly reduced, in keeping with the elevation of RV. The increase in RV may amount to 35% between the ages of 20 and 60[8]. In part this is related to weaker respiratory muscles, increased stiffness of the rib cage and changes in the thoracic spine which together prevent air being 'squeezed out'[3], but this is compounded by the fall in elastic recoil of the lungs. Because pleural pressure at the lung bases is less negative than at the apices at low lung volumes, there is less pressure acting on small airways to keep them open and in the lung bases they tend to close. With age-associated loss of recoil forces, pleural pressures are further compromised and the smaller airways close at higher lung volumes, again starting in the lower parts of the lungs when the subject is erect. This process may be exacerbated by a tendency of the airways to become more compliant with age[9].

Airway conductance

Although structural changes such as calcification of cartilage do occur in the large airways as ageing progresses, this appears to be of little physiological significance.

Transfer factor for carbon monoxide

Between the ages of 30 and 65, TLCO falls by approximately 19% in non-smoking men and women[10]. Until recently it was considered possible to separate the transfer factor into a membrane component and a volume component – the pulmonary capillary blood volume – but doubt has now been cast upon the validity of the calculations of membrane component[11]. Our present understanding of TLCO is that it represents the volume of haemoglobin accessible to the alveolar air. Where the transfer properties of the alveolar membrane and those of the red cells have been calculated by the method of Roughton and Forster[12], however, one sees a fall in the membrane component with age with little reduction in the pulmonary capillary blood volume[13]. The explanation may lie in the enlargement of alveolar ducts and

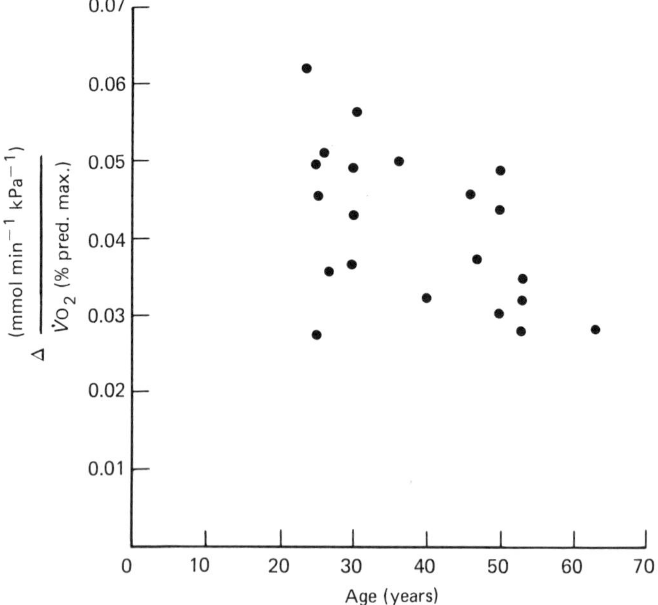

Figure 1.6 Rise in TLCO on exertion (ΔTLCO/ΔV_{O_2}) plotted against age in 20 healthy subjects (correlation coefficient $r = -0.50$)

respiratory bronchioles that takes place with ageing which is accompanied by a reduction in the amount of alveolar walls and alveolar parenchyma[14], causing a loss of alveolar–capillary surface area.

Interestingly, the ability of the pulmonary capillary bed to expand with exertion – important for the oxygenation of the red cell as it traverses the pulmonary capillary and hence for maintenance of arterial oxygen tension on exercise – does not diminish with age. Figure 1.6 shows that the slope of the rise of TLCO on exertion correlates poorly with age[15]. This observation supports the view that the functional pulmonary capillary blood volume is relatively unaffected by the ageing process.

We may now compare the flow-volume loop of the 30-year-old man shown earlier (Figure 1.3) with the loop he is likely to exhibit at the age of 65 (Figure 1.7). There is a change in shape of the expiratory curve with increasing convexity at lower lung volumes, a slight reduction in peak expiratory flow rate (PEFR) and FEV_1 with a smaller fall in FVC and a concomitant rise in RV. VA is reduced in sympathy with the rise in RV but TLCO shows a relatively greater fall. The airway conductance (SGAW) shows little or no change.

Clinical application

How applicable is this battery of lung function tests to the average elderly patient? In a personal series, 47 out of 50 subjects aged up to 75 years and with preserved higher mental function managed the whole sequence. After 75 years of age, the proportions satisfactorily completing these investigations declined, so that only 9 out of 20 in the 75–85 years age range, and 1 out of 10 persons in the over 85 age range, provided meaningful data. If spirometry only is attempted, the latter figures improve to 14 out of 20 and 3 out of 10 respectively. Thus with careful instruction and adequate rehearsal of the manoeuvres, most patients should be able to furnish readings for FEV_1, FVC and PEFR.

If an elderly patient is unable to perform the single breath TLCO manoeuvre owing to inability to hold the breath for 10 s, a rebreathing method may be used. This involves rebreathing a standard gas mixture from a bag of known volume over a certain period of time. Calculated rebreathing values of TLCO have a linear relationship to single breath values. The procedure is relatively simple for the subject and has the added advantage of being applicable to breathless patients who cannot hold their breath[16].

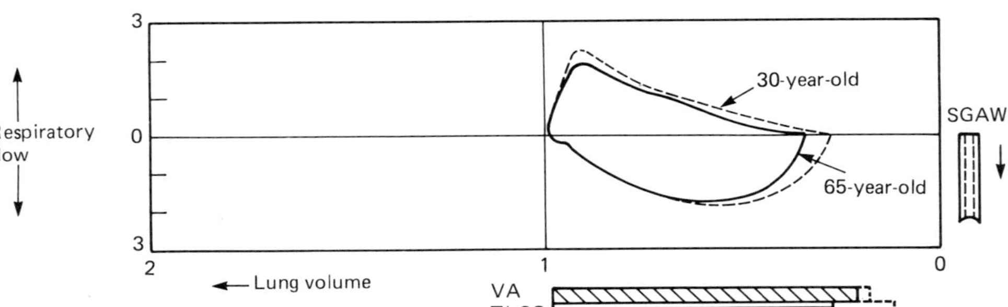

Figure 1.7 Lung function characteristics of a 30-year-old man (as in Figure 1.3) and like characteristics at the age of 65

Arterial blood gas measurements are simple to perform and give some index of the efficiency of gas exchange. Although ageing has little influence on the arterial carbon dioxide tension or arterial pH, arterial oxygen tension (Pao_2) falls as ageing progresses so that our 65-year-old will have a value nearly 10 mmHg (1.3 kPa) less than the 30-year-old[5]. The reduction in Pao_2 is matched by an increase in the alveolar–arterial oxygen tension difference. The deterioration in these variables is due to mismatching of ventilation and perfusion in the lungs as age advances. Airway closure at lung bases in the elderly breathing at the tidal volume range will cause inspired gas to go to apical areas where perfusion is relatively poor, and conversely the basal areas will have better perfusion but poor ventilation.

Exercise arterial blood gas measurements are particularly useful in the patient who complains of breathlessness or fatigue on exertion but is unable to perform standard pulmonary function tests. Physical work, such as walking down a hospital corridor, stresses the lungs and can augment resting functional derangements or even detect those not found at rest. Healthy people do not desaturate on exercising but patients with lung disease, such as chronic airway obstruction or pulmonary fibrosis, commonly do so. Figure 1.8 shows exercise profiles of two groups of patients with chronic airflow obstruction. Group I, whose mean age was 67 years, had emphysema clinically and demonstrated significant hypoxaemia on exercise, whereas those in group II (mean age 65) with chronic bronchitis tended to maintain their arterial oxygen tension. This finding, in part, is due to the very low TLCO values of the emphysema patients compared to those of the chronic bronchitics (33% and 76% predicted respectively).

Clinical inspection of a patient's chest radiograph, permits some judgement on the size of the lungs. In fact, very accurate measurements of TLC are recordable by radiography[17]. To do this, the volume of the chest is calculated and the volume of non-lung structures is subtracted; estimates of whole lung volume are very close to those of gas dilution or plethysmography. Although at present limited to specialist centres, this technique may be of considerable value.

In conclusion, the ageing process is responsible for decline in respiratory function, although this may not be as great as was previously thought. The impairment in lung function does reduce the efficiency of the lungs and their functional reserve; this will not, however, compromise an individual's daily activities. With the increase in descriptive work on pulmonary function throughout the world, we are learning more about the effects of ageing on

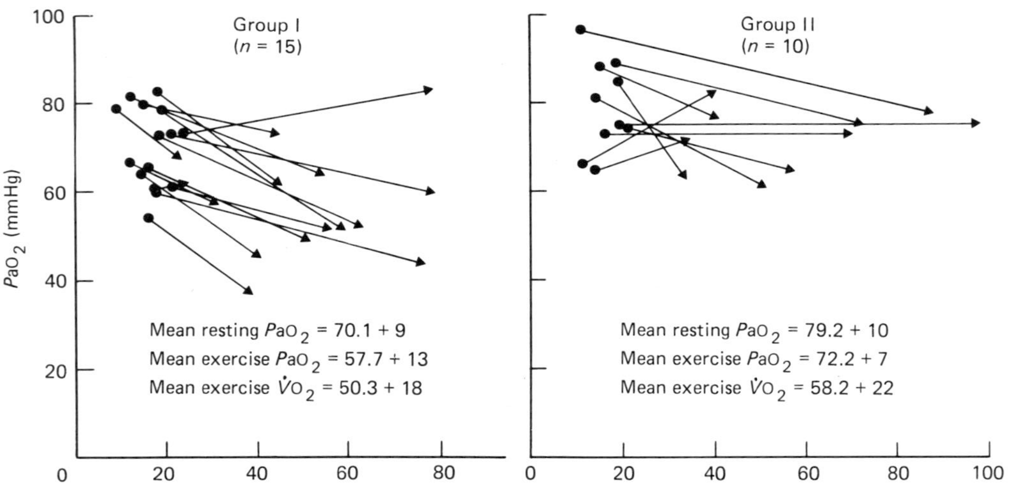

Figure 1.8 Effects of progressive exercise on arterial oxygen tension in 15 patients with emphysema (Group I, mean age 67) and 10 patients with chronic bronchitis (Group II, mean age 65)

12

physiological variables. There are no shortcuts to testing lung function in the elderly and we should all be encouraged to use standard methods of testing as a minimum, if only to allow for easy comparison with previous studies and to encourage uniformity in standards for those embarking on longitudinal research.

Acknowledgements

The data presented in Figures 1.1–1.4, 1.6 and 1.8 were obtained at the Lung Function Unit, Brompton Hospital. I would like to acknowledge the assistance of the technical staff and thank Professor D. M. Denison for his advice.

References

1. DAVIES, N. J. H. *Br. J. Dis. Chest,* **76**, 105 (1982)
2. DENISON, J., LAW, M., AL-HILLAWI, H. and GEDDES, D. In *Cigarettes and the Lung* (ed. G. Cumming and G. Bonsignore), Plenum Press, New York (1984)
3. GIBSON, G. J., PRIDE, N. B., O'CAIN, C. and QUAGLIATO, R. *J. Appl. Physiol.,* **41**, 20 (1976)
4. KRUMPE, P. E., KNUDSON, R. J., PARSONS, G. and REISER, K. *Clin. Geriat. Med.,* **1**, 143 (1985)
5. COTES, J. E. *Lung Function: Assessment and Application in Medicine,* 3rd edn, Blackwell Scientific, Oxford (1975)
6. BURROWS, B., LEBOWITZ, M. D., CAMILLI, G. E. and KNUDSON, R. J. *Am. Rev. Resp. Dis.,* **133**, 974 (1986)
7. LEINER, G. C., ABRAMOWITZ, S., SMALL, M. J. *et al. Am. Rev. Resp. Dis.,* **88**, 644 (1963)
8. BATES, D. V., MACKLEM, P. T. and CHRISTIE, R. V. *Respiratory Function in Disease,* 2nd edn, Saunders, London (1971)
9. KNUDSON, R. J., CLARK, D. F., KENNEDY, T. C. and KNUDSON, D. E. *J. Appl. Physiol.,* **43**, 1054 (1977)
10. CRAPO, R. O. and MORRIS, A. H. *Am. Rev. Resp. Dis.,* **123**, 185 (1981)
11. FORSTER, R. E. *Thorax,* **38**, 1 (1983)
12. ROUGHTON, F. J. W. and FORSTER, R. E. *J. Appl. Physiol.,* **11**, 290 (1957)
13. HAMER, N. A. J. *Clin. Sci.,* **23**, 85 (1962)
14. THURLBECK, W. M. and ANGUS, G. E. *Chest,* **67**, 35 (1975)
15. AL-HILLAWI, A. H., CRAMER, D., BUSH, A. and DENISON, D. (in press)
16. AL-HILLAWI, A. H., CRAMER, D. and DENISON, D. M. *Thorax,* **40**, 236 (1984)
17. DENISON, D. M., PIERCE, R. J. and WALLER, J. F. *Br. J. Dis. Chest,* **75**, 371 (1981)

Chapter 2

The clinical significance of bronchial hyperreactivity

M. K. Benson

A characteristic feature of patients with asthma is the development of airway narrowing in response to a variety of extrinsic stimuli. This phenomenon can be documented by using various bronchial provocation tests to demonstrate the degree of bronchial reactivity (airway responsiveness)[1]. The stimuli applied are generally non-specific in that they will provoke a response in any patient with asthma. This differs from specific allergic responses occurring in atopic individuals. This latter type of challenge will not be considered further.

The basic test involves applying a stimulus to the airways, usually by inhalation and measuring the physiological response which reflects a change in airway calibre. Although it is generally assumed that bronchospasm is the major end organ response, development of mucosal oedema and intraluminal mucus may also be contributory factors.

Bronchial challenge tests have been variously used:

1. As a clinical diagnostic test.
2. In examining the pathophysiology of asthma.
3. In evaluating the use of therapeutic agents.
4. In epidemiological surveys.

This paper will concentrate on the practical aspects of performing bronchial challenge tests and examine their usefulness in clinical diagnosis.

Measuring bronchial reactivity

Quantitative measurement of bronchial reactivity requires accurate documentation of the applied stimulus as well as the physiological response. Studies have varied widely in both these respects. The types of stimuli that have been used are listed in Table 2.1. They can be divided into those having an irritant effect operating through a reflex arc and those with specific pharmacological actions. The latter may have direct effects on bronchial

Table 2.1 Non-specific bronchoconstrictor stimuli

Pharmacological stimuli	*Irritant stimuli*
Histamine	Exercise
Methacholine	Cold air
Prostaglandin F_2 alpha	Fog
Leukotrienes C_4 and D_4	Sulphur dioxide
Adenosine	Distilled water

muscle as well as indirect effects via mediator release or through irritant receptors. When using inhaled stimuli, a number of delivery systems have been used and this makes comparisons between studies difficult[2–4].

Measurement of the physiological response usually depends on tests of forced expiration, such as the forced expiratory volume in one second (FEV_1) or the peak expiratory flow rate (PEFR). Airway resistance changes may be used when anticipating only small fluctuations, but the fact that it is more difficult to perform limits its clinical usefulness. In considering some of these practical aspects, attention will be focused on two of the more commonly used tests, namely the exercise provocation test and the dose-response curve to inhaled histamine.

Exercise challenge test

Exercise-induced asthma is a well-recognized clinical entity. Formal testing requires a period of continuous running for 6 min sufficient to make the patient moderately breathless and produce a heart rate of approximately 150/min[5]. Although a treadmill is required for accurate standardization, free range running is acceptable and more likely to produce an asthmatic response. The mechanism of exercise-induced asthma is related to a cooling and drying of the bronchial mucosa since the response can be reduced when the subject inhales warm, moist air[6]. Thus atmospheric conditions will influence the end response.

The pattern of response is illustrated in Figure 2.1, whereby PEFR is recorded before, during and after exercise. A small increase in peak flow during exercise occurs in most normal and asthmatic subjects. Any fall in peak flow is likely to develop within 5 min of ceasing exercise. The interpretation of the result has limitations. Normal subjects show a decline of less than 10% in peak flow, although some asthmatic subjects also fall within this

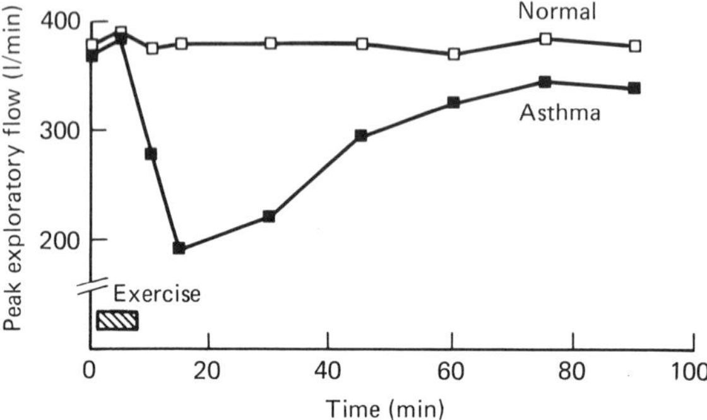

Figure 2.1 Response to 6 min exercise test in normal subject and patient with exercise-induced asthma

range. Decreases of greater than 15% make the diagnosis of asthma virtually certain.

The limitations of exercise testing in an elderly population are obvious. Many patients will be unable to perform the sustained exercise necessary for the test because of other illness or limited mobility. In clinical practice, the test is usually confined to children and young adults who have symptoms suggestive of asthma, but who have normal lung function at the time of study.

Histamine dose-response curve

Many different methods have been used for inhalation provocation tests with inhaled histamine. Early studies tended to use 'single dose' challenges, but more recently dose-response curves have been used. The basic principle of the histamine dose-response test is to deliver increasing concentrations of nebulized histamine solution to the bronchi until a defined physiological end point is reached (Figure 2.2). Variability in response can be due to either biological or technical factors. Care needs to be taken to minimize the latter. Factors that result in biological variability need to be recognized and taken into account when interpreting results.

The simplest method utilizes a timed period of tidal breathing from a continuous output nebulizer. When using the method of Cockcroft *et al.*[4], the challenge is delivered for 2 min with a 5 min interval between successive challenges. This time interval is important since it will determine whether the dose-response relationship is cumulative or non-cumulative. With a 5 min interval between challenges, there is no significant cumulative effect. Any

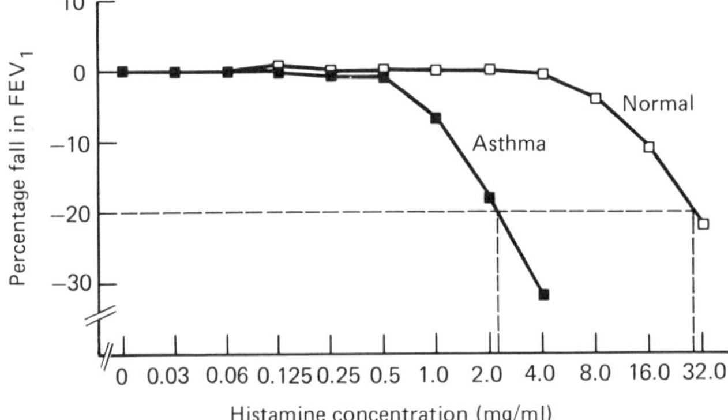

Figure 2.2 Dose-response curve to inhaled histamine in normal subject and patient with moderate severe asthma. The derived histamine PC_{20} is respectively 24 mg/ml and 2.2 mg/ml

bronchoconstrictor response is evident 1 min after the challenge has been delivered. The concentration of histamine is doubled for each successive challenge until a fall in FEV_1 of greater than 20% has been achieved. The result is expressed as the concentration of histamine which will produce a 20% fall in the FEV_1 (the histamine PC_{20}).

Interpretation of results

As with most biological variables, bronchial reactivity is not an all-or-nothing response. There is a spectrum of responses ranging from normal subjects, who do not bronchoconstrict to relatively high concentrations, to asthmatic patients exhibiting marked bronchial hyperreactivity. Most normal subjects have a histamine PC_{20} greater than 16 mg/ml whereas symptomatic asthmatics may respond to concentrations as low as 0.03 mg/ml[7].

Increases in bronchial reactivity are not limited to patients with asthma but have been recorded in individuals with allergic rhinitis[8], chronic obstructive airway disease[9] and cystic fibrosis. Before considering these different diagnostic groups, it is important to recognize that other biological factors can result in changes in reactivity within any individual. Factors that modify reactivity include recent use of medications[10], exposure to sensitizing agents and allergens[11], respiratory tract infections[12] and the baseline airway calibre[13].

The administration of bronchodilators immediately prior to bronchial challenge will reduce the end organ response. Single doses of inhaled steroids or sodium cromoglycate have no blocking effect on inhaled histamine, but regular prophylactic treatment will result in a reduction in reactivity[14]. This improvement is probably due to an alteration in the background level of inflammatory mediators, which serve to augment the response to non-specific stimuli. Conversely, prior exposure to allergens or a recent respiratory tract infection will result in an increase in bronchial reactivity.

Clinical diagnosis

From the diagnostic viewpoint, the main consideration is whether bronchial provocation tests can be helpful in distinguishing patients with asthma from normal subjects or from patients with other respiratory diseases. Patients with mild asthma, without current symptoms, may have a modest increase in reactivity although there will be some overlap with normal subjects and with patients with allergic rhinitis. Those patients who are symptomatic will have greater increases in reactivity. It is in this group of patients, who have normal lung function and atypical presenting symptoms, that challenge tests may be of some value. In patients with classic asthma, there is a strong positive correlation between the degree of bronchial reactivity and asthma severity.

One factor that complicates interpretation of results is the baseline airway calibre. Empirically, airway calibre should affect bronchial reactivity since in airways already narrowed, a small further reduction in calibre will result in a disproportionately greater physiological change. This relationship has been demonstrated in patients with asthma and chronic obstructive airway disease whereby those individuals with more severe obstruction are likely to be more responsive. It should be stressed that this is not the only or even most important factor since many patients with normal lung function do have increased bronchial reactivity. Its relevance becomes more important in the determination of changes in reactivity seen in patients with chronic obstructive airway disease.

In many middle-aged and elderly patients presenting with breathlessness and evidence of airway obstruction, the clinical uncertainty lies in whether their problem is due to asthma or irreversible airway obstruction. There is little comparative data in patients with established airway obstruction on the diagnostic value of challenge testing and in practice measuring the response to a bronchodilator is safer and more appropriate. There is some evidence that individuals with the greatest bronchodilator responsiveness will also show the greatest degree of reactivity to a constrictor stimulus[14].

Conclusions

Bronchial provocation testing is relatively simple and dose-response curves provide reproducible measurements of bronchial reactivity. In general, subjects showing increased reactivity to one form of bronchial challenge will also have increased responses to other constrictor stimuli.

In patients with symptoms suggestive of asthma, but with normal lung function, bronchial challenge testing may be diagnostically useful.

In patients with established asthma, the degree of bronchial reactivity will correlate with the severity of asthma as assessed by other means, such as diary cards, regular peak flow measurements or treatment requirements.

In patients with established airway obstruction, the response to a bronchodilator is safer and of equal diagnostic value.

References

1. HARGREAVE, F. E., RYAN, G., THOMPSON, N. C. *et al. J. All. Clin. Immunol.*, **68**, 347–355 (1981)
2. CHAI, H., FARR, R. S., FROEHLICH, L. A. *et al. J. All. Clin. Immunol.*, **56**, 323–327 (1975)
3. YAN, S. K., SALOME, C. and WOOLCOCK, A. J. *Thorax*, **38**, 760–765 (1983)
4. COCKCROFT, D. W., KILLIAN, D. N., MELLON, J. J. A. *et al. Clin. All.*, **7**, 235–243 (1977)
5. JONES, R. S., WHARTON, M. J. and BUSTON, M. K. *Arch. Dis. Childh.*, **38**, 972–977 (1963)
6. STRAUSS, R. H., McFADDEN, E. R., INGRAM, R. H. *et al. J. Clin. Invest.*, **61**, 433–440 (1978)
7. COCKCROFT, D. W., BERSCHEID, B. A., MURDOCK, K. Y. *et al. J. All. Clin. Immunol.*, **75**, 142 (1985)
8. TOWNLEY, R. G., RYO, U. Y., KALOTKIN, B. M. *et al. J. All. Clin. Immunol.*, **56**, 429–442 (1975)
9. RAMSDALE, E. H., MORRIS, M. M., ROBERTS, R. S. *et al. Thorax*, **39**, 912–918 (1984)
10. COCKCROFT, D. W., KILLIAN, D. N., MELLON, J. A. *et al. Thorax*, **32**, 429–437 (1977)
11. HARGREAVE, F. E. and DOLOVICH, J. In *Asthma: Physiology, Immunopharmacology and Treatment* (ed. A. B. Kay, K. F. Austen and L. M. Lichtenstein), Academic Press, London, ch. 16, pp. 263–275 (1984)
12. EMPEY, D. W., LAITENEN, L. A., GOLD, W. M. *et al. Am. Rev. Resp. Dis.*, **113**, 131–139 (1976)
13. BENSON, M. K. *Br. J. Dis. Chest*, **69**, 227–239 (1975)
14. COCKCROFT, D. W. *Ann. All.*, **55**, 527–534 (1985)
15. BENSON, M. K. *Thorax*, **331**, 211–213 (1978)

Chapter 3

Nephrology and the older patient

J. M. Bone

Introduction

The difficulties in delivering nephrological care to older patients arise from at least three different factors. First, facilities and numbers of doctors in the United Kingdom are inadequate to meet the need. Secondly, nephrology is poorly taught in medical schools, and few geriatricians will have had much more than a glimpse of the subject. Thirdly, the chronological age of the patient is a poor guide to the biological age which will determine likely benefit from intensive and costly therapies.

Renal services are expanding, and more specialists are being recruited and trained. This article will try to improve understanding of the problems faced by the older patient with impaired renal function, and outline the services available. However the third, conceptual problem should be considered by geriatricians themselves, and with some urgency.

Topics considered will include: how disordered renal function induces disease in the patient; the special problems faced by the

Table 3.1 Some important functions of the kidney

Excretion
    Nitrogenous waste: urea, creatinine, uric acid, 'others'
    Salts: sulphate, phosphate
    Drugs: digoxin, aminohexose antibiotics
    Surplus nutrients: water, sodium, potassium etc.

Regulation
    Water and electrolytes

Metabolic
    Renin/angiotensin/aldosterone
    Erythropoietin
    Vitamin D
    Clearance of insulin, calcitonin, parathyroid hormone, β_2-microglobulin

older patient; the services available; some ethical points; and some possible solutions.

Renal function and renal failure

The kidney has excretory, regulatory and metabolic functions (Table 3.1) that are variably affected as renal failure progresses. Likewise, treatment of end-stage disease can only replace these functions to a variable extent, despite great technological advances. It is in the context of the older patient that the limitations of therapy must be specially appreciated.

Excretion

Nitrogenous waste
Urea, uric acid and creatinine are all examples of end metabolites cleared by the kidney. Urea is derived from breakdown of proteins, and both exogenous and endogenous factors can affect its rate of production. While a reduction in dietary protein intake can spare the kidney from 'the labour of elimination' of this substance, and reduce its plasma concentration, the value of such a measure seems proved only in patients with very advanced disease. Protein restriction results in a decreased production of sulphuric acid from sulphydryl groups in the amino acids methionine, cysteine and cystine. There is also a reduction in phosphate absorbed from the gastrointestinal tract since many proteinaceous foods contain this mineral in abundance. Some benefits of dietary intervention may result from these other metabolic changes, rather than from the reduction in urea production, as originally thought.

Creatinine is synthesized in muscle at a fairly constant rate. Its excretion by the kidney is largely by glomerular filtration, with a small contribution from tubular secretion. In practical terms the creatinine clearance often changes in line with the glomerular filtration rate (GFR) and can provide a useful measure of renal function. Furthermore, in adults with a stable muscle mass, the relative constancy of creatinine production means that the reciprocal of the plasma concentration changes in proportion to the creatinine clearance (and GFR), as follows:

$$\text{GFR} \propto \text{creatinine clearance} = \frac{U\text{cr} \times V}{P\text{cr}} = \frac{\text{Constant}}{P\text{cr}} \propto 1/P\text{cr}$$

where $U\text{cr}$, $P\text{cr}$ are the creatinine concentrations in urine and plasma, and V the volume of urine produced in unit time.

One advantage of this manipulation arises from the clinical observation that in many renal disorders GFR declines steadily with time. Thus a simple plot of $1/P$cr can be used to estimate the rate of progression into renal failure. Treatment can be evaluated and the need for dialysis and transplantation forecast (Figure 3.1).

In the elderly, however, certain limitations to the interpretation of plasma urea and creatinine concentrations must be borne in mind. Often dietary protein will be poor and muscle mass reduced and so the rise in plasma urea and creatinine levels in renal failure will be reduced. Measurement of creatinine clearance using 24-hour urine collections can overcome this difficulty, and in addition yield important information on nutritional state. For example, the urea excretion rate closely follows the dietary protein intake. The urinary sodium and potassium excretion rates also reflect dietary habits and can be measured on the same sample. In the untrained patient, however, collection errors are common. Nevertheless, for many patients the additional discipline of bringing to clinic regularly their carefully timed output from the previous day presents no real hardship and may encourage compliance with other measures.

Uric acid concentrations rise only as renal failure advances, since tubular secretion predominates and can compensate for a reduction in GFR. Gout is uncommon, and the role of allopurinol uncertain. Allopurinol itself is excreted by the kidney, and the dosage should be reduced in renal failure.

While urea, creatinine and uric acid may be relatively innocuous, other nitrogenous substances, including guanidines, amines and oligopeptides of around 1000 daltons molecular weight, accumulate as well. These other substances may have more to do with the pathogenesis of the syndrome of uraemia.

Inorganic salts

Sulphate arises from oxidation of certain amino acids, as already mentioned, and phosphate is absorbed from the intestine. Both accumulate in renal failure, and contribute to the 'anion gap'. Phosphate may have a pathogenetic role through precipitation

Figure 3.1 *(opposite)* Reciprocal serum creatinine plots against time (note different scales and units). (*a*) Patient with bilateral renal atrophy following obstructive uropathy. Date of dialysis (May 1988) predicted from intercept of extrapolated regression with $1/P$cr $= 1.0$ l/mmol, when Pcr $= 1000\,\mu$mol/l. (*b*) Membranoproliferative glomerulonephritis. Hypertension finally controlled March 1987, with reduction in rate of progression. (*c*) Progressive membranous glomerulonephritis treated successfully in December 1985, with pulse intravenous methylprednisolone followed by oral prednisolone and azathioprine

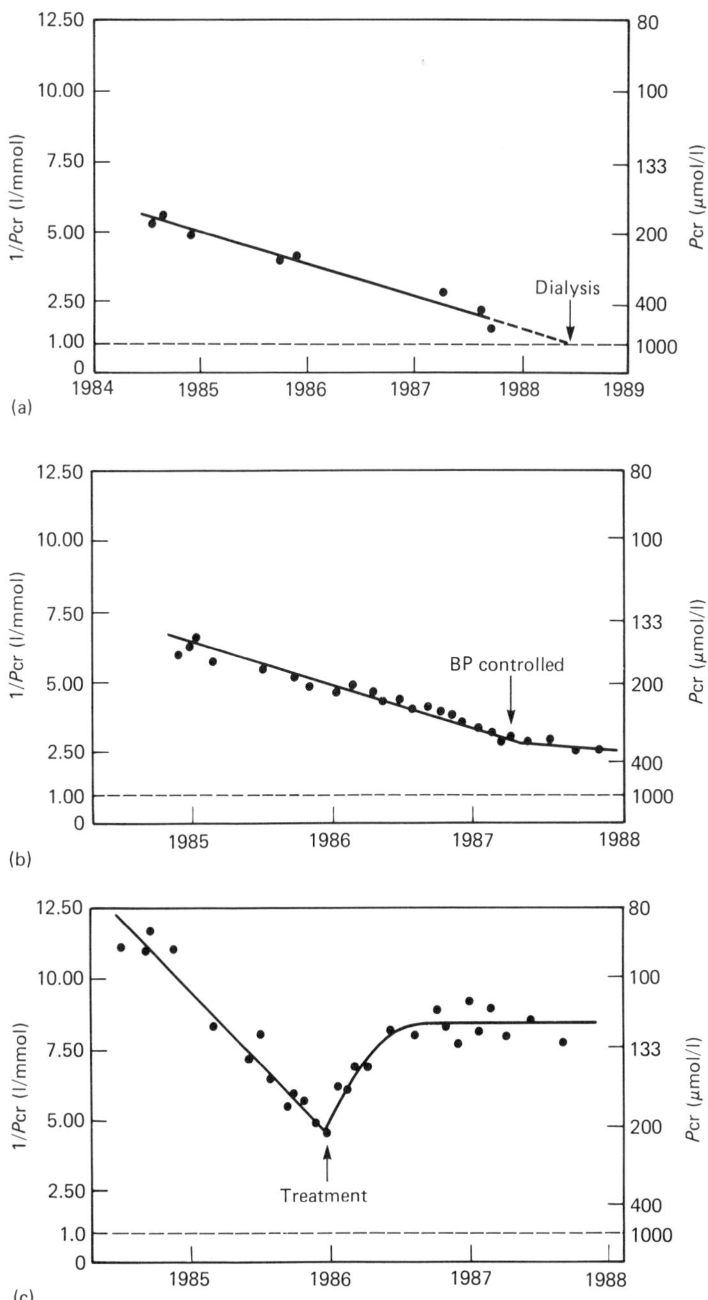

12.50
10.00
7.50
5.00
2.50
1.00
0
1/Pcr (l/mmol)
80
100
133
200
400
1000
Pcr (μmol/l)
Dialysis
1984 1985 1986 1987 1988 1989
(a)

12.50
10.00
7.50
5.00
2.50
1.00
0
1/Pcr (l/mmol)
80
100
133
200
400
1000
Pcr (μmol/l)
BP controlled
1985 1986 1987 1988
(b)

12.50
10.00
7.50
5.00
2.50
1.0
0
1/Pcr (l/mmol)
80
100
133
200
400
1000
Pcr (μmol/l)
Treatment
1985 1986 1987 1988
(c)

with calcium in skin and other tissues, including the kidney, causing pruritus, and accelerated progression to renal failure. A reduction in plasma ionized calcium as phosphate concentrations rise may provoke secondary hyperparathyroidism.

Drugs

Many drugs are excreted by the kidney but almost all of these are either eliminated by the liver or metabolized to less active forms. The two groups of drugs that must be watched with great caution are digoxin and its congeners, and the aminohexose antibiotics. The dosage of digoxin should be reduced but not the frequency of administration. By contrast, for amikacin, tobramycin and gentamicin the dosage is usually unaltered, but the frequency reduced in proportion to the degree of renal failure. For both drug groups, levels should always be monitored.

Surplus nutrients

Many nutrients are consumed regularly in excess of requirements, simply to allow us to get what we want from food, namely sufficient energy to sustain our daily activities. While starch stores in grains and tubers provide a dietary source of energy, other components of plants (and of animals) are ingested at the same time. Thus, intracellular minerals such as magnesium, potassium and phosphate, which are not required to any extent in healthy adult life, are absorbed and need to be excreted. Salt added for preservation and taste is usually unnecessary in such quantities unless excessive loss has been caused by disease. Water is taken socially, and as an inevitable accompaniment of alcohol, given the synthetic limitations of yeast and the high price of spirits. In kidney failure dietetic measures may thus be helpful, but hunger and social difficulties often result.

Regulation

The kidney maintains homeostasis of the body fluids, their volume and mineral composition by a variety of mechanisms. Many surplus nutrients require conservation from time to time. In early renal failure, the inability to conserve water causes nocturia and provokes thirst and polydipsia. A failure of sodium conservation can arise in a number of disorders, including chronic pyelonephritis. This can be recognized clinically in a patient with advanced renal disease who has an unduly low blood pressure and no oedema. Sometimes salt supplements can improve renal function and delay the need for renal replacement.

It is worth noting that in many patients the regulatory mechanisms themselves allow damaged kidneys to compensate for the loss of tissue. Normally, enormous quantities of water (approximately 150 litres daily) and solutes are filtered from the plasma and almost all reabsorbed by the tubules. This means that only a small adjustment in tubular function is needed to balance the effects of even very advanced disease. For example, the urine in health contains less than 0.5% of the water and sodium that have been filtered by the glomeruli. As renal failure progresses, a reduction in tubular reabsorption from 99.5% to 97.5% would allow a fivefold increase (from 0.5% to 2.5%) in the proportion excreted by the remaining nephrons. In this way a fivefold reduction in nephron mass, equivalent to a loss of 80% in GFR, could be sustained with no overall effect on salt and water balance.

Similar adjustments in tubular reabsorption and secretion allow homeostasis to be more or less maintained with respect to potassium, magnesium, phosphate and hydrogen ions.

Metabolism

The kidney plays a central role in the renin/angiotensin/aldosterone regulation of blood pressure, sodium and potassium balance. In renal failure, however, hypertension most commonly arises from an increase in plasma volume following severe reduction in GFR, and renin has little influence. The system is none the less important, since an increase in the tubular secretion of potassium by the remaining nephrons, mediated by aldosterone, maintains the plasma concentration within normal limits until renal failure is far advanced. Dangerous hyperkalaemia can result from inhibition of the angiotensin converting enzyme by captopril or enalapril, or from inhibition of the effect of aldosterone by spironolactone. Agents such as triamterene that act more directly on the distal nephron are often contraindicated. Lack of erythropoietin plays a large part in the anaemia of chronic renal failure.

Insulin, parathyroid hormone, calcitonin and β2-microglobulin are peptides cleared primarily by glomerular filtration. In consequence they too can accumulate as renal failure progresses. The clinical significance in diabetics arises from their decreasing requirement for exogenous insulin as end-stage renal disease approaches. In patients who have been treated by haemodialysis for many years β_2-microglobulin can form amyloid deposits. This causes arthropathy and carpal tunnel syndrome, and may result in autonomic neuropathy or cardiac failure.

The kidney still seems to be the major source of 1,25-dihydroxy vitamin D. Deficiency of this active metabolite results in osteo-malacia and secondary hyperparathyroidism. The ensuing lesion of renal osteodystrophy causes bone pain, deformity and patho-logical fractures, and can present in some patients even after successful transplantation.

Clinical features of renal disease

In many respects, the clinical features in renal failure can be inferred from the effects of the progressive loss of the functions already described.

In chronic renal failure, tiredness can arise from the anaemia. Polyuria, nocturia and thirst result from the failure to conserve water. Ankle swelling is a consequence of sodium retention, and headaches follow if hypertension develops. These are all non-specific features which can also suggest disease of other major organ systems. Often they occur late, when more than 80–90% of the renal reserve has been lost, since the regulatory capacity of the tubules allows compensation over a relatively wide range.

When less than 10% remains, however, and the creatinine clearance has fallen below 10 ml/min, other features of the uraemic syndrome develop. These may include nausea, vomiting, haemor-rhagic colitis, peripheral and autonomic neuropathy, twitching and convulsions, impaired immunity, pericarditis and depressed platelet function, as well as the other more predictable features discussed above.

Acute and chronic renal failure

In physiological terms the differences between acute and chronic renal failure do not greatly affect the changes that develop, but there are obviously differences in the rate at which they appear. In acute renal failure oliguria or anuria may be the presenting feature, rather than the final event. Hyperkalaemia is common and life-threatening because there is no time for adaptation, and the little residual function that remains after a gross insult from hypotensive infection or trauma is easily overwhelmed by greatly increased metabolic demands.

Much that follows relates primarily to the patient with chronic renal disease. However, many of the principles and some of the ethical considerations apply with equal force to those with acute renal failure.

Physiological aspects of treatment

Conservative

Treatment by conservative measures can begin early in the course of chronic renal disease. Control of blood pressure is normally achieved with two drugs or less, but sometimes more than three are needed. Plasma phosphate can be reduced by giving aluminium hydroxide, magnesium and calcium salts by mouth to prevent intestinal absorption of phosphate. Metabolic acidosis is controlled with sodium bicarbonate. In different clinical circumstances either dietary salt restriction or the opposite, a supplement to the oral salt intake, may be needed. A low protein diet can help uraemic symptoms at a later stage.

The artificial kidney

Haemodialysis   As should be fairly common knowledge today, in the haemodialysis process blood, usually drawn from an arterio-venous fistula in the forearm, is circulated through a dialyser, where a synthetic membrane allows diffusion of nitrogenous wastes and unwanted salts into the dialysis fluid, made by a kidney machine. The kidney machine, which is a very expensive piece of equipment, prepares the fluid from tap water and a concentrated solution of salts, then heats and tests it to ensure that the electrolyte concentration is similar to plasma water. Other electronic monitors are needed to protect the extracorporeal circuit. Water and sodium are removed by ultrafiltration down a hydrostatic pressure gradient which can be adjusted to the needs of the patient. Usually three treatments lasting 4 hours each are needed weekly, and strict dietary discipline with respect to salt and water is also required since the patient, between treatments, is essentially anephric.

Peritoneal dialysis   Here the blood in the peritoneal capillaries is separated from the dialysis fluid by the natural peritoneal membrane. The principle is the same as in haemodialysis, but water and sodium are removed by an osmotic pressure gradient, usually achieved by incorporating glucose into the dialysis fluid. The process is less efficient, and can take 10 hours three times weekly for the same effect.

A variant, continuous ambulatory peritoneal dialysis (CAPD), has become very popular in recent years. Some 2 litres of dialysis fluid are run into the peritoneal cavity through an indwelling Silastic cannula, and left to equilibrate for 6–8 hours before being drained and replaced with a fresh exchange. The process is repeated throughout the day, week, month and year. In consequence fluid and salts are removed continuously, and dietary measures can be less stringent.

All peritoneal dialysis fluid must be sterile, and peritonitis is an ever-present risk unless strict asepsis is practised at all times.

Haemofiltration   This relatively new technique employs an extra-corporeal circuit, like haemodialysis, but the membrane in the dialyser or haemofilter is much more permeable to water and solutes. With only a small hydrostatic pressure gradient, large volumes of fluid containing the unwanted uraemic waste can be removed from the plasma by filtration and replaced by an idealized sterile solution. For reasons that are poorly understood, this procedure is tolerated by older patients better than haemodialysis, even when treatment times are similar.

Renal metabolic replacement   Not surprisingly, the artificial kidney plays no synthetic metabolic role. However, the essential renal step in vitamin D metabolism may be bypassed pharmacologically by giving 1-alpha-hydroxy vitamin D. This congener of vitamin D is already hydroxylated at the 'kidney' position. In the liver the 25-hydroxyl group is added, and the result is indistinguishable from the 'natural' product. Also 1,25-dihydroxy vitamin D is itself available. Both active metabolites increase absorption of phosphate as well as calcium from the gastrointestinal tract, and this can be very dangerous in patients held on conservative treatment before dialysis becomes necessary. As explained earlier, in patients with moderately severe renal failure, further accelerated decline in renal function can be provoked by deposition of calcium phosphate salts in the renal parenchyma. This can occur even when plasma levels appear satisfactory. For patients on dialysis, however, there is usually no major reservation over the use of active vitamin D metabolites, providing plasma chemistries are monitored closely.

Human erythropoietin, now synthesized using recombinant DNA technology, is now under clinical trial, and promises relief from symptoms of anaemia.

Peptides of middle molecular weight are not cleared well through the standard artificial kidney, but even β_2-microglobulin is cleared with newer, more permeable membranes.

Special problems with older patients

My own perception of the special problems facing older patients with renal disease is shown in Table 3.2.

Table 3.2 Special problems with older patients

More systemic disease	More drugs
Cardiovascular	Diuretics
Cerebrovascular	Non-steroidal anti-inflammatory drugs
Respiratory	Angiotensin converting enzyme inhibitors
Neoplasia	
Locomotor	'Senile' nephrosclerosis
Dementia	
	Autonomic neuropathy
More doctors	
Conflicting advice	Social
Missing case sheets	Mobility
	Family help
	Loss of role
	Personal hygiene

Systemic disease

Major systemic disease must determine a worse prognosis on dialysis or after transplantation, and a poorer quality of life. These considerations will also affect the cost-benefit analysis of intensive care of older patients with acute renal failure. In this context, however, recovery of renal function is usually complete, as long as the patient survives the acute illness, and the renal costs in the long term are insignificant.

Chronic renal replacement therapy carries its own symptomatology. This is not tolerated so well by patients already suffering from partial failure of other organ systems. In addition, a certain amount of agility is needed for patients to look after themselves on dialysis.

Neoplasia

Malignant neoplasms contraindicate transplantation within at least one year of successful removal, since steroids and immunosuppressives can activate undetected metastases.

Drugs and doctors

More systemic disease results in more drugs being prescribed by more doctors. It is not unusual for patients to attend several clinics in the same hospital, for general surgery, orthopaedics, dermatology as well as nephrology and geriatrics. Case sheets can be permanently in transit, followed at an unsafe interval by laboratory reports or letters which never, quite, get to their destination. Drugs prescribed by the renal team are sometimes stopped or altered by others with no background understanding. For example, in renal failure aluminium hydroxide is used as a phosphate binder, and it makes little sense to replace it with an H2-antagonist, or to discontinue treatment when gastrointestinal symptoms settle. Likewise, diuretics may be prescribed by nephrologists in alarmingly high dosage with no apparent concern over potassium supplementation. As explained earlier, drugs that inhibit angiotensin converting enzymes, as well as spironolactone and triamterene, can cause hyperkalaemia in chronic renal failure by interfering with distal tubular homeostatic mechanisms.

By contrast, diuretics given even in low dosage can provoke acute renal failure through salt depletion, since patients disabled through cerebrovascular disease, or arthritis, may not be able to sustain their normal dietary intake. In gastroenteritis, too, there is often an increased salt loss from the bowel as well as a reduced oral intake. None the less, diuretics may continue to be taken on 'doctor's orders'.

Non-steroidal anti-inflammatory drugs can cause an interstitial nephritis, as well as papillary necrosis. The spectrum of disease ranges from a salt-losing state with a low blood pressure to severe chronic renal failure and hypertension. A common pathogenetic factor may be the inhibition of prostaglandin synthesis and the loss of an important protective mechanism against renal ischaemia.

'Senile' nephrosclerosis

Demographic studies show that in man there is a slow but steady loss of renal function with age. In the ageing rat, death from renal failure is common, often with hypertension and heavy proteinuria. By contrast most humans die from other disorders, albeit with some loss of renal reserve. Furthermore, while hypertension is seen more commonly in the elderly, heavy proteinuria is normally caused by some other primary or secondary glomerular disorder, for example membranous glomerulonephritis, diabetes or amyloidosis. It is difficult clinically to separate senile nephrosclerosis from the effects of hypertension, prostatic obstruction, degenerative vascular disease or years of analgesics.

Autonomic neuropathy

Autonomic neuropathy develops in chronic renal failure as part of the uraemic syndrome. Its effects are augmented in diabetes and amyloidosis. Patients with postural hypotension tolerate haemodialysis poorly, since there is no reflex compensation for the rapid reduction in plasma volume when fluid is removed, and the blood pressure falls to symptomatic levels. Peritoneal dialysis, which is slower, may be better for such patients, but overall prognosis is still poor.

Social factors

The social factors listed in Table 3.2 relate not only to quality of life, but also to the ability of patients to look after themselves on dialysis, and be supported if they have difficulties. The significance of these considerations will be discussed below.

Services available

Table 3.3 lists services available for the older patient.

Table 3.3 Services available for older patients

Conservative
   Outpatient clinics
   Inpatient consultation

Replacement
   Continuous ambulatory peritoneal dialysis (CAPD)

   Haemodialysis:
     hospital
     staffed satellite
     home

   Transplantation:
     cadaveric
     living relative

Conservative

Increasingly, nephrologists welcome early referral for the diagnosis and, hopefully, intervention that may delay the need for expensive therapies or avoid them altogether. Specialist advice is normally needed for blood pressure control, salt and water balance, and other measures that will optimize conservative management. Older patients can experience most of the nephropathies affecting younger patients. Renal biopsy is often more hazardous, but the increased risks have to be balanced not only against the dangers of blind therapy with steroids in high dosage, and other powerful immunosuppressives, but also against the chances of kidney failure if a reversible lesion is wrongly diagnosed. Rapidly progressive crescentic glomerulonephritis, renal polyarteritis nodosa and progressive membranous glomerulonephritis can now be treated successfully, and the need for dialysis averted.

Dialysis

Hitherto, dialysis policies in the United Kingdom have been orientated towards treatment at home with full responsibility taken by the patient, supported by close relatives, and with minimal involvement by trained nursing staff. By contrast, in other European countries and in the United States, hospital dialysis or staffed satellite dialysis has been developed to a greater extent, and in consequence older patients are treated with greater ease. The use of CAPD from 1978 provided an obvious outlet for older patients in the United Kingdom, but the vulnerability of this group soon became apparent. The symptomatology of dialysis is more evident in the elderly, and deserves separate consideration.

Haemodialysis
Vascular access   Blood is usually taken from an arteriovenous fistula in the forearm. Atherosclerosis can reduce the flow in the distal radial artery and the fistula is correspondingly poor. The next procedure is usually to move proximally to the antecubital fossa, and then to the other forearm. Thus several visits to theatre for both patient and struggling surgeon may be needed. Poor arterial flow increases the risks of distal ischaemia from steal through the fistula, and venous gangrene is not uncommon.

Two large calibre needles are used for each dialysis, three times weekly. Although local anaesthetic is often used, needle phobia can impede rehabilitation.

Time   Time is spent not only on dialysis, but also in preparing the machine and extracorporeal circuit before the treatment and clearing up afterwards. Travel to and from the unit can be prolonged if ambulance services are under pressure. Thus treatment can take many hours of the patient's time each week. This may be a reasonable investment for a younger patient awaiting early transplantation and with many years to live. For the elderly it may seem too high a price to pay.

Self dialysis   Self dialysis is encouraged in many units. Patients generally take a pride in the acquisition of new skills. Self-sufficiency, too, promotes compliance in other directions, such as dietary discipline between dialysis and subsequently taking regular medications after transplantation. An older, infirm, or frankly disabled patient may be unable to respond to pressures to become as independent as younger patients on the unit, and frustration and disappointment can result.

Hypotension   Hypotension on dialysis, as fluid is removed, is seen more frequently in older patients since they often have less cardiac reserve. Autonomic neuropathy can also contribute to this distressing symptom.

Post-dialysis morbidity   Many patients feel tired and listless for some hours after dialysis. This is tolerated more readily by the young but may add to the burden of an older patient.

Anaemia   Anaemia persists and contributes to the diminished cardiac reserve.

Effects on the family   Effects on the home environment are not insignificant. These may be felt even when patients are treated in hospital or at a satellite unit, in view of the time spent away from the family. In addition, the older patient on dialysis is normally more disabled by his renal disease and its treatment.

Peritoneal dialysis
Peritoneal dialysis and especially CAPD corrects the biochemical abnormalities and removes fluid much more gently than haemodialysis. In consequence, hypotension on dialysis and the morbidity afterwards do not occur. In addition, there are no problems over vascular access, and no needle phobia. Other difficulties arise, however, especially for the elderly.

Peritonitis   Peritonitis is a perpetual risk, especially in CAPD where the lines between the peritoneal cannula and the bags containing the sterile dialysis fluid are interrupted 28 times each week. Patients with poor personal hygiene, who have not grasped the importance of an utterly strict aseptic technique, will be particularly vulnerable.

Hernia   Inguinal hernia presents a special problem for patients on CAPD, and may be more prevalent as age advances, through weakness of the muscles of the anterior abdominal wall. With 2 litres of additional fluid in the peritoneal cavity, other potential spaces will be filled. Thus hernial sacs will expand to accommodate the hydrostatic pressure.

Diverticular disease   Peritonitis with mixed organisms strongly suggests perforation of a colonic diverticulum. Older patients are more likely to experience this complication, which usually signifies the need to change the mode of dialysis therapy.

Backache   Backache in patients on CAPD arises from the unaccustomed load of carrying extra weight in front of the midline, in the form of the 2 litres of dialysis fluid.

Self dialysis   As with patients on haemodialysis, the pressure to take full responsibility for treatment and to learn new skills may be too much to expect from the elderly. In addition, there is often little or no support for treatment at home. Failure is expensive since central facilities are occupied to an increasing extent. Frustration and disappointment are common.

Anaemia   Anaemia is less severe than in patients on haemodialysis, but may still contribute to morbidity.

From the foregoing it may seem that a patient must be fit, both mentally and physically, to survive and benefit from dialysis treatment. None the less, there are still many older patients who can enjoy an extension of life in this manner, and even be candidates for transplantation. In recent months on Merseyside and in North Wales, out of 100 patients starting dialysis as many as 33 were over 60 years old, and of these 12 were over 70. While many still need medical and nursing support on hospital dialysis (as outpatients), a significant number are undergoing dialysis with acceptable independence at home or in minimally staffed satellite units. Moreover, one 64-year-old woman has already been transplanted successfully.

Transplantation

Patients must be fit for surgery, not only on one occasion, but sometimes for two or three further visits to the operating theatre if complications arise or the graft has to be removed. They must be able to tolerate aggressive immunosuppression with prednisolone, azathioprine, cyclosporin A and antilymphocyte globulin. Thus good nutrition and adequate dialysis are essential for safe transplantation.

An older patient may be more likely to die from acute myocardial infarction shortly after the operation. Strokes are not uncommon in the first year: this may result from a rise in the haematocrit and a recovery of platelet function.

None the less, as in younger patients, kidney transplantation offers benefits that cannot be matched by dialysis. The results have improved enormously with better tissue matching and immuno-suppression and with pre-transplant blood transfusions which appear to induce a state of specific immunological unresponsive-ness. In many units cadaveric graft survival exceeds 75% after 3 years. Results are even better if a living relative can offer a kidney, but this is less likely in the older patient.

Ethical considerations

Questions that are often asked include:

1. Can the impoverished health service afford expensive renal replacement therapies for older patients who will benefit less and die sooner from systemic disease of other major organs?
2. Should cadaveric kidneys be used for the elderly when younger patients are waiting on dialysis?

There are several answers that can be given to both questions. First, a greater proportion of older patients are dialysed and even transplanted in other developed countries of Europe and America. There is no evidence that older patients 'benefit less' than younger. Moreover, costs of dialysis are lower than the costs of providing long-term care for the incapacitated elderly, or indeed the costs of maintaining a younger person in prison for social or criminal misbehaviour. Transplantation is cheaper than dialysis, and offers a better quality of life.

It should also be said that survival and quality of life may even be better in some older patients than younger diabetics or patients with systemic disease, who are now accepted as candidates for replacement therapy. Moreover, in younger patients compliance with dietary restrictions on dialysis can be poor. In such patients failure to take immunosuppressives can account for unnecessary graft loss and wastage of kidneys that have been harvested and transplanted, at considerable expense, both emotional and finan-cial. Older patients are often more compliant. Also tissue-matching criteria are drawn up to optimize the use of cadaveric kidneys and to minimize wastage. Moreover, a younger patient is more likely to be offered a kidney from a living relative.

Finally, in answer to our two questions, we might say that an older patient might expect a greater reward for contributions to society made throughout a full working lifetime.

Biological age

An important consideration relates to the 'biological age' of the patient. If this could be evaluated it should offer a better assessment of comparative benefit and expectation of life than chronological age. At present, clinical evaluation is based on general experience of morbidity and mortality. Patients are screened on the way to the nephrologist by the family practitioner, a physician, urologists and geriatricians whose perception of the problems and resources may be more or less well informed. Often the best assessment can be made by the nephrologist from serial clinic visits when shortcomings in cardiopulmonary reserve, in the ability to comply with treatment and in the depth of family support will be revealed.

Solutions

Possible solutions to the problems I have discussed are summarized in Table 3.4. Geriatricians need more training in nephrology, and nephrologists in geriatrics. Computer storage of biochemical

Table 3.4 Solutions to the problems

Nephro-geriatricians
Computerization
More: staffed dialysis
       transplants
       money
An index of biological age

data and other information has helped greatly on my own unit, when case sheets cannot be found. Because of the greater dependence of the older patient, more support on dialysis will be needed. Patients should be encouraged to take responsibility for their own treatment, but more time should be allowed. The argument over whether younger patients should be given preference for kidney transplantation would vanish if there were more grafts available. What is needed, in nephrological as in other medical interventions, is some more precise measure of a patient's biological age rather than his or her chronological age. Biological age would be an index of reserve capacity, and hence ability to respond to physiological and biochemical challenge and thus provide a more objective and equitable prediction of outcome of treatment.

Chapter 4

Interventional cardiology and cardiac surgery in the elderly

O. J. M. Ormerod and S. Westaby

Introduction

Cardiovascular disease is the commonest cause of death in the elderly[1] and in an increasingly aged population there will be an ever larger number of subjects with heart disease presenting for treatment. Cardiac surgical procedures with cardiopulmonary bypass, or the more recently developed percutaneous alternatives, may be appropriate in many elderly individuals. However, these procedures carry a substantial fatality and morbidity in this age group and, moreover, they are very expensive. It is important, therefore, for physicians and surgeons involved with the elderly, to consider carefully the benefits and limitations of these techniques, so as to give informed advice to their patients and to make best use of the resources.

The term 'elderly' is deliberately vague. Chronological age is often unhelpful in the assessment of an individual. Some patients are young for their years and others age prematurely. Physiological age[2], taking account of general health and 'vigour'[3], is more useful. In the past two decades, with increasingly safe cardiac surgery, being 'elderly' has advanced by ten years, from 60 years[4] to a generally accepted 70 years in the 1980s.

The description 'elderly' begs some questions: not least is what separates them from the young? For practical purposes the elderly present with pathologies that they have brought with them from middle years[5]. Do the elderly respond differently to cardiac surgery, in terms of fatality, morbidity and symptomatic improvement? There are no randomized trials of cardiac surgery in the elderly but there is a substantial body of literature addressing these questions. We will review the literature relating to coronary bypass surgery, valve replacement, percutaneous transluminal coronary angioplasty and balloon valvuloplasty in the elderly.

Coronary artery bypass surgery

Fatality – technical factors

In the past 20 years the risks of cardiac surgery with cardiopulmonary bypass have decreased considerably. This is particularly so in the elderly. Smith *et al.*[6] reported a series of 157 patients, aged 65 years or older, operated on between 1960 and 1976. Of these, 47 patients underwent coronary artery bypass grafting (CABG) with a fatality of 19.1%, which was only slightly less than for valvular surgery (22.6%). The method of myocardial protection was not stated but the authors emphasized, amongst other factors, the importance of the techniques of cardiopulmonary bypass. This point is well illustrated by Meyer *et al.*[7], reporting on 95 patients aged 70 years or more, undergoing CABG between 1969 and 1974. Initially their technique consisted of anoxic cardiac arrest (simply cross-clamping the aorta until the heart became still). Their overall fatality was 22.1%. However, in 1974 they changed their technique to intermittent cross-clamping for distal anastomoses, performing the proximal anastomoses with a beating heart, thus minimizing myocardial ischaemic time. The fatality for their final 21 patients was substantially lower at 4.8%.

Technical advances, such as the now almost standard systemic hypothermia, topical cold irrigation of the pericardium and cold hyperkalaemic cardioplegic arrest, have resulted in a consistently lower fatality of 1–6%[8–14] in selected elderly patients (Table 4.1). In addition to improved myocardial protection, the practice of more complete myocardial revascularization[15] may have contributed to the reduction in fatality and perioperative myocardial infarction.

Table 4.1 Hospital fatality among patients undergoing CABG in eight published series

Fatality (%)			
Elderly	Young	Period	Series
19.1		1960–1976	Smith *et al.* [6]
22.1		1969–1974	Meyer *et al.* [7]
6.0	0.8	1975	McCallister *et al.* [16]
5.0	2.5	1978–1980	Hibler *et al.* [11]
5.8	2.8	1970–1981	Elayda *et al.* [12]
5.2		1974–1979	Gersh *et al.* [1]
2.7	0.4	1978–1983	Montague *et al.* [13]
5.9	1.9	1981–1984	Rose *et al.* [14]

Fatality – patient factors

While the chances of an elderly patient surviving cardiac surgery have improved, a persisting fatality of around 5% for selected patients remains substantial when compared to an overall fatality of 1–2% for younger patients[13,16] (Table 4.1). The increased fatality in the elderly is consistent in other series in which authors compare their experience with younger patients[9,11], but most series are too small to detect factors other than age that may be contributing. Elderly patients are likely to have more chronic disease and present later in the natural history with more extensive disease, poorer left ventricular (LV) function and more often as an emergency[9]. Data from the Collaborative Study in Coronary Artery Surgery (CASS) have been analysed to address this question[17]. Pooled data on 6630 patients undergoing CABG, of all ages and from 15 centres contributing to the registry, revealed a greater operative fatality with increasing age, female sex, impaired global and regional wall motion and emergency, or to a lesser extent urgent, in contrast to elective surgery. More detailed analysis of the CASS registry in patients of 65 years or older ($n =$ 1086)[1] suggested increasing fatality with age; also more severe coronary disease, impaired LV function and associated medical conditions.

Montague *et al.*[13] report a large series (597) of patients of 70 years or more with a hospital fatality rate of 2.7% compared with 0.4% for 4125 patients of less than 70 years. Their findings supported the CASS data with fatality increased in those patients older than 80 years of age, with evolving infarction, coexistent illness, major LV dysfunction and emergency operation.

An alternative approach to studying the influence of severity of disease and age has been adopted by Hockberg *et al.*[18], who matched 75 subjects aged 70 or more with 75 younger controls for sex ratio, previous myocardial infarction (MI), unstable angina and preoperative balloon pumping. Patients were similar in respect of symptomatic state, severity of disease and grafts inserted. The fatality in the older group was three times that in the younger, although, perhaps because of small numbers, this difference was not statistically significant. No comment was made concerning the severity of LV dysfunction, although the relatively low mean LV end diastolic pressure would suggest that LV function may have been reasonably good in both groups.

Data from the CASS registry[17] suggested that female patients of all ages had a higher fatality. Faro *et al.*[19] reported a much greater fatality in women than in men (28.6% as against 6%,

P<0.002) in 105 patients more than 70 years old operated on between 1974 and 1980. In a more recent study Rose *et al.*[14], studying 201 patients aged 70 years or more having CABG between 1981 and 1984 also found a higher fatality in women (8.8% versus 4.8%), although again, perhaps because of small numbers, this was not statistically significant. The influence of female sex was investigated in 102 elderly women having CABG between 1978 and 1983 by Jeffery *et al.*[20]. These patients were compared to male controls matched for age, LV ejection fraction, incidence of unstable angina and number of grafts. No difference in hospital fatality was found, although women suffered a significantly increased incidence of recurrent 'angina-like chest pain'.

Complications

Improvements in myocardial protection and more complete revascularization have reduced not only the fatality of CABG but also the incidence of non-fatal myocardial complications such as low cardiac output state and perioperative MI. Using principally anoxic arrest in 1969–1974, Meyer *et al.*[7] recorded a 26% (25/95) incidence of myocardial complications. In contrast, Rose *et al.*, in a 1981–1984 series, found an incidence of low cardiac output of 0% and perioperative MI of 4.1% in 1242 patients aged less then 70 years but 7.9% in 201 patients aged 70 years or more[14]. Whilst the incidence of perioperative MI has fallen, it remains high in elderly compared with younger patients. This reflects the difficulty in achieving complete revascularization in subjects with chronic, severe and diffuse disease.

The incidence of non-cardiac morbidity, especially cerebral events, remains high in old compared with younger patients. Kuan *et al.*[21], in a series of 365 consecutive CABG patients of all ages, found a 20% incidence of major complications in patients aged over 60. Additional risk factors were prolonged cardiopulmonary bypass and diabetes mellitus. Rose *et al.*[14] could find no relation between surgical morbidity and the severity of coronary disease, angina or LV function, whereas Montague *et al.*[13] found the probability of morbidity to be related to the presence of peripheral vascular disease, urgent/emergency operation and concomitant illness. Knapp *et al.*[9] reported significantly more strokes and psychosis in old than in younger patients. Patients with aortic calcification were particularly at risk of stroke, suggesting that this complication may be caused by debris released from the wall of the aorta on applying or releasing the cross-clamp. The incidence of stroke remains 2–4%[10,13,14,22], with a further 2–17% incidence of transient psychosis or confusion[9,10,13].

Follow-up

Most series comment that survivors show a marked symptomatic improvement, at least in the short term[8,23,24]. Rahimtoola *et al.*[25] followed 1304 patients undergoing CABG between 1974 and 1984, who were aged 65 or more at the time of operation, for up to 10 years. These were compared to patients aged less than 65 years. Operative fatality was similar (3% versus 2% respectively). Survival was lower in the older patients compared with both the younger patients and the predicted life expectancy of the general population. There was no difference, however, in the incidence of recurrent angina.

The CABG patients aged 65 and over in the CASS registry[26] were followed for 5 years. Survival was significantly less than in younger subjects (83% versus 91%, $P<0.0001$) and survival decreased with increasing age ($P<0.04$). Survival was also influenced by severity of global and regional LV impairment and associated medical conditions, but not the extent of coronary disease. Event-free survival and actuarial recurrence of angina were better than among younger patients, presumably because of higher death rates in the more severely afflicted and lower physical activity of older patients. Actuarial recurrence of angina was higher in women than men.

Comparison with medical treatment

There are no randomized comparisons of medical versus surgical treatment for the elderly. However, the CASS registry may help[27]. Of 1491 patients entered into the CASS registry between 1974 and 1979, excluding those with left main stenosis and angiographic deaths, 861 underwent surgery with an operative fatality of 4.6% and 630 patients were treated medically initially, although 11% subsequently underwent surgery for symptomatic reasons. At follow-up of up to 4.4 years, 62% of surgical patients were free of chest pain compared with 29% of medically treated patients. However, the number of Class I and II (mild to moderate) medical patients had increased from 40% to 84%. Statistical analysis (Cox proportional-hazards model) suggested an independent effect of surgery on survival ($P<0.0001$). This benefit of surgery was greatest in the high-risk patients. There was no difference in survival in low-risk patients treated medically or surgically. As in randomized studies in younger patients, improvement in survival associated with surgery was seen particularly in patients with extensive coronary disease.

Interpretation of these data is limited by the major differences in important baseline characteristics of the two groups. Whilst surgical patients had more severe symptoms, medically treated patients had a substantially higher incidence of poor LV function, a factor known to have a potent influence on survival in both medically and surgically treated groups. Statistically adjusted curves, for what they are worth, still showed a significantly better survival at 6 years in the surgical group (79% versus 64%, $P<0.0001$) although less than in the raw data. However, it must be emphasized that the surgical group was highly selected. It seems likely that the patients at high risk of surgical complications were treated medically. Thus the surgical high-risk group may have been at lower long-term risk than many of the medical group.

Cost and resources

The high frequency of morbidity in the elderly might be expected to prolong intensive care and hospital stay. Series that report hospital stay confirm this[13,14,25,28,29]. Roberts *et al.*[30] comment that this expense may be worthwhile in severely symptomatic patients as they will subsequently use fewer medical resources than if left without operation. Elayda *et al.*[12] consider all the elderly to be at high risk (fatality 4.7%) and only operate if medical therapy has failed.

Summary

Technical improvements in myocardial protection have substantially reduced operative mortality and morbidity in CABG. More complete revascularization has probably contributed but is likely to be particularly important in improved long-term results. The preoperative extent of coronary disease as such is only important in long-term survival or recurrence of angina if complete revascularization is not achieved. This may explain the poorer results in women, who tend to have more diffuse disease and technically more difficult vessels to graft than men. Clearly the surgical suitability of coronary vessels is central to patient selection.

The influence of the severity of antecedent LV damage on surgical results, in general, is undoubtedly important. The exact extent of this influence is difficult to judge in these uncontrolled, highly selected series when LV function would have been a major consideration in opting for surgery in these elderly patients.

The purely economic argument that the use of surgical resources is justified by a subsequent reduction in the chronic burden on medical and social services would only be true if patients selected for surgery were to have a high chance of a satisfactory and sustained surgical result.

Valvular surgery

As in coronary bypass surgery, there has been a steady reduction in the risk of cardiac valve replacement from an operative fatality of 17.5–20% in the 1960s[4,31] to 4.3–7% with improved myocardial protection[33–35]. The risk in isolated aortic valve replacement (AVR) may be very low[36], although it is probably still higher than in younger patients[37] even when matched for preoperative LV function and sex[38]. The fatality of mitral valve replacement (MVR) is higher than AVR[36] and may be very high (23%) if there is severe haemodynamic disturbance, particularly resulting in functional tricuspid reflux[39]. As in the younger age group with valve disease, more late deaths can be expected compared with CABG[35,40], presumably owing to irreversible myocardial damage, but long-term survivors can expect a satisfactory symptomatic improvement[33,37] similar to younger patients[40] and life expectancy returns to close to normal[39,41].

The fatality of double valve replacement in the elderly is high, ranging from 15% to 33%[4,36], although the numbers reported are very small.

Two series make the observation that the fatality of valve replacement plus CABG differs little from that of isolated valve surgery[41] and may even be lower[38]. This is in sharp contrast with experience in younger patients. No satisfactory explanation can be found for this curious paradox; perhaps it is a sampling phenomenon as the numbers are rather small.

The complication rate among the elderly is appreciable[38], with both stroke and perioperative MI occurring more frequently than in younger patients (CVA 5.2% versus 2.8%; MI 4.4% versus 3.2%; $P<0.05$). However, this may be related to the degree of vascular disease rather than to the valvular disease. Craver *et al.*[41] found an increased risk of stroke and postoperative confusion in the elderly only in the group undergoing valve replacement and CABG. In this series 64% of patients (98/152) underwent isolated AVR; no patient suffered a stroke.

Percutaneous interventions

Coronary angioplasty

Percutaneous transluminal coronary angioplasty (PTCA) is now widely practised and experience with elderly patients is accumulating. Early pooled data from the National Institutes Angioplasty Register suggested a higher fatality, complication rate and primary failure rate (inability to achieve adequate dilatation) and difficulty in crossing the stenosis in elderly patients[42], particularly women[43]. This may reflect more severe disease, with technically more difficult lesions in the women[44]. More recent data, particularly from more experienced centres, suggest that primary success rate and long-term improvement are similar in elderly and younger patients[45]. PTCA offers an alternative to CABG, although producing less improvement in symptoms[46], and is likely to be a useful palliative treatment for patients with severe symptoms unsuitable for cardiopulmonary bypass surgery[47].

Balloon valvuloplasty

The use of balloon catheters has been established in paediatric cardiology for many years. Balloon valvuloplasty attempting to dilate calcified, stenotic aortic valves in the elderly was first described by Cribier *et al.* in 1986[48]. Initial attempts were undertaken in the post-mortem room or perioperatively[49–51]. It appears that dilatation may be achieved by fracturing a valve leaflet along its base to form a 'hinge'. Investigators were reassured that potentially embolic material would not be dislodged and the procedure was taken into the catheter laboratory. Early experience would suggest a reasonable primary success rate and a low fatality, considering the morbid state of some of the early subjects[50]. Morbidity has been considerable, with difficult haemostasis at the entry site and temporally related stroke[50]. Both these complications reflect the potential problems of placing, and removing, a very large catheter in the femoral artery and manoeuvring it up a tortuous and atheromatous aorta. Such complications may be reduced with improvements in the technology of the balloons and introducers. Symptomatic improvement has been encouraging[50], but the time-course of long-term recurrence of the stenosis remains to be assessed.

Balloon valvuloplasty may prove to be a useful alternative to cardiopulmonary bypass surgery in severely ill patients, those with intercurrent illness, severe independent coronary disease or the very elderly who are unsuitable for valve replacement.

General comments and conclusions

Selected elderly patients may undergo cardiopulmonary bypass with acceptable surgical risk and with an expectation of prolonged symptomatic improvement. It is equally true that many are at high risk or have a disappointing surgical result. Therefore the selection of candidates for surgery is of paramount importance.

Despite the high incidence of symptomatic coronary disease in the elderly, CABG is a relatively unusual form of treatment in this age group. Even in the larger American series[12,45] patients aged more than 70 comprise only about 10% of the annual bypass grafting workload, suggesting that those coming to surgery were highly selected. The fatality and morbidity figures discussed here probably approach the best current surgery can achieve.

It is easy to envisage how the addition of unfavourable coronary vessels, impaired LV function, atheroma of the aorta and associated medical conditions could raise the surgical risk to a disqualifying extent. Even in an intermediate risk group, the increased operative fatality and risk of recurrent angina may outweigh the improved life expectancy and symptomatic state of survivors. Whilst life should always be valued, absolute life expectancy is, perhaps, less of an overwhelming consideration for an older person than is quality of life. It is perhaps all the more important to avoid a failed operation, with an early recurrence of angina or, worse still, a chronically disabling stroke. Thus the temptation to operate on the high-risk patient with severe angina on the grounds that they have little to lose by attempted surgery with only a low likelihood of a sustained improvement in symptoms, should be resisted.

The place of aortic valve replacement for symptomatic, isolated aortic stenosis is secure in most age groups as medical treatment is ineffective and surgery carries a low risk. Mitral valve replacement in the elderly is more difficult to justify as the natural history is longer and less predictable, medical palliation is more successful and surgery carries a significantly higher risk. Similarly the presence of independent coronary disease increases both morbidity and possibly fatality and will limit the success of surgical correction of the valve lesion. Double valve disease is likely to be associated with considerable myocardial damage and the risks of surgery may be unacceptable in the elderly.

Percutaneous interventions for both coronary disease and aortic stenosis in the elderly may provide a less expensive and risky alternative to the management of patients less able to tolerate thoracotomy.

It is accepted that a patient should not be refused surgery on the basis of age alone. However, patients over the age of 70 years, and particularly women, should be carefully selected and operations offered to those with severe angina despite full medical therapy but with favourable coronary vessels, good LV function and an absence of significant medical conditions; those with the lowest risk and best chance of a long-term improvement with surgery.

References

1. GERSH, B. J., KRONMAL, R. A., FRYE, R. L. *et al.* Coronary arteriography and coronary artery bypass surgery. Mortality and morbidity in patients aged 65 years and older. A report from the Coronary Artery Surgery Study. *Circulation,* **67**, 483–491 (1983)
2. GANN, D., COLIN, C., HILDNER, F. J. *et al.* Coronary artery bypass surgery in patients seventy years of age and older. *J. Thorac. Cardiovasc. Surg.,* **73**, 237–241 (1977)
3. TAYLOR, J. G., RABINOVICH, E., MIKELL, F. L. *et al.* Percutaneous transluminal coronary angioplasty as palliation for patients considered poor surgical candidates. *Am. Heart J.,* **111**, 840–844 (1986)
4. AHMAD, A. and STARR, A. Valve replacement in geriatric patients. *Br. Heart J.,* **31**, 322–326 (1969)
5. POMERANCE, A. Cardiac pathology in the elderly. In *Geriatric Cardiology* (ed. R. J. Noble), *Cardiovascular Clinics,* Davis, Philadelphia, pp. 9–49 (1981)
6. SMITH, J. M., LINDSAY, W. G., LILLEHEI, R. C. and NICOLOFF, D. M. Cardiac surgery in geriatric patients. *Surgery,* **80**, 443–448 (1976)
7. MEYER, J., WUKASCH, D. C., SEYBOLD-EPTING, W. *et al.* Coronary artery bypass in patients over 70 years of age. *Am. J. Cardiol.,* **36**, 342–345 (1975)
8. DuCAILAR, C., CHAITMAN, B. R. and CASTONGUAY, Y. Risks and benefits of aortocoronary bypass surgery in patients aged 65 or more. *Can. Med. Assoc. J.,* **122**, 771–774 (1980)
9. KNAPP, W. S., DOUGLAS, J. S., CRAVER, J. M. *et al.* Efficacy of coronary artery bypass grafting in elderly patients with coronary artery disease. *Am. J. Cardiol.,* **47**, 923–930 (1981)
10. BERRY, B. E., ACREE, P. W., DAVIS, D. J. *et al.* Coronary bypass operations in septuagenarians. *Ann. Thorac. Surg.,* **31**, 310–313 (1981)
11. HIBLER, B. A., WRIGHT, J. O., WRIGHT, C. B. *et al.* Coronary bypass surgery in the elderly. *Arch. Surg.,* **118**, 402–404 (1983)
12. ELAYDA, M. A., HALL, R. J., GRAY, A. G. *et al.* Coronary revascularization in the elderly. *J. Am. Coll. Cardiol.,* **3**, 1398–1402 (1984)
13. MONTAGUE, N. T., KOUCHOUKAS, N. T. and WILSON, T. A. S. Morbidity and mortality of coronary bypass grafting in patients 70 years of age and older. *Ann. Thorac. Surg.,* **39**, 552–557 (1985)
14. ROSE, D. M., GELBFISH, J., JACOBOWITZ, I. T. *et al.* Analysis of morbidity and mortality in patients 70 years of age and over undergoing isolated coronary bypass surgery. *Am. Heart J.,* **110**, 341–346 (1985)
15. KIRKLIN, J. W., KOUCHOUKAS, N. T., BLACKSTONE, E. H. and OBERMAN, A. Research related to surgical treatment of coronary artery disease. *Circulation,* **60**, 1613–1618 (1979)
16. McCALLISTER, B. D., SCHMEIDT, M. and REED, W. A. Coronary artery bypass in patients over the age of 70: initial and late results. *Circulation,* **52**, Suppl. II, p. 91 (1975)

17. KENNEDY, J. W., KAISAR, G. C., FISHER, L. D. *et al.* Clinical and angiographic predictors of operative mortality from Collaborative Study in Coronary Artery Surgery (CASS). *Circulation,* **63**, 793–802 (1981)

18. HOCKBERG, M. S., LEVINE, F. H., DAGGETT, W. M. *et al.* Isolated coronary artery bypass grafting in patients seventy years of age and older. Early and late results. *J. Thorac. Cardiovasc. Surg.,* **84**, 219–223 (1982)

19. FARO, R. S., GOLDEN, M. D., JAVID, H. *et al.* Coronary revascularization in septuagenarians. *J. Thorac. Cardiovasc. Surg.,* **86**, 616–620 (1983)

20. JEFFERY, D. L., VIJAYANAGAR, R. R., BOGNOLO, D. A. and ECKSTEIN, P. F. Results of coronary artery bypass surgery in elderly women. *Ann. Thorac. Surg.,* **42**, 550–553 (1986)

21. KUAN, P., BERNSTEIN, S. B. and ELLESTAD, M. H. Coronary bypass surgery morbidity. *J. Am. Coll. Cardiol.,* **3**, 1391–1397 (1984)

22. ENNALBI, K. and PELLETIA, L. Morbidity and mortality of coronary artery surgery after the age of 70 years. *Ann. Thorac. Surg.,* **42**, 197–200 (1986)

23. HIGGINBOTHAM, M., HUNT, D., WHITE, A. and CLAREBROUGH, J. Surgical treatment of angina pectoris in the elderly. *Med. J. Aust.,* **2**, 664–666 (1981)

24. ASHOR, G. W., MEYER, B. W., LINDISMITH, G. G. *et al.* Coronary artery disease. Surgery in 100 patients 65 years of age and older. *Arch. Surg.,* **107**, 30–33 (1973)

25. RAHIMTOOLA, S. H., GRUNKEMEIER, G. L. and STARR, A. Ten year survival after coronary bypass surgery for angina in patients 65 years and older. *Circulation,* **74**, 509–517 (1986)

26. GERSH, B. J., KRONMAL, R. A., SCHAFF, H. V. *et al.* Long term (5 year) results of coronary bypass surgery in patients 65 years old or older: a report from the Coronary Artery Surgery Study. *Circulation,* **68**, Suppl. II, pp. 190–199 (1983)

27. GERSH, B. J., KRONMAL, R. A., SCHAFF, H. V. *et al.* Comparison of coronary bypass surgery and medical therapy in patients 65 years of age and older. A non-randomised study from the coronary artery surgery study (CASS) Registry. *N. Engl. J. Med.,* **313**, 217–224 (1985)

28. RICH, M. W., SANDZA, J. G., KLEIGER, R. E. and CONNORS, J. P. Cardiac operations in patients over 80 years of age. *J. Thorac. Cardiovasc. Surg.,* **90**, 56–60 (1985)

29. PELLETIA, L. C., CASTONGUAY, Y. R. and CHAITMAN, B. R. Open heart surgery in elderly patients. *Can. Med. Assoc. J.,* **128**, 409–412 (1983)

30. ROBERTS, A. J., WOODHALL, D. D., CONTI, C. R. *et al.* Mortality, morbidity and cost-accounting related to coronary artery bypass grafting in the elderly. *Ann. Thorac. Surg.,* **39**, 426–432 (1985)

31. AUSTIN, W. G., DeSANCTIS, R. W., BUCKLEY, M. J. *et al.* Surgical management of aortic valve disease in the elderly. *JAMA,* **211**, 624–626 (1970)

32. DeBONO, A. H. B., ENGLISH, T. A. H. and MILSTEIN, B. B. Heart valve replacement in the elderly. *Br. Med. J.,* **2**, 917–919 (1978)

33. COMMERFORD, P. J., CURCIO, A., ALBANESE, M. and BECK, W. Aortic valve replacement in the elderly. *S. Afr. Med. J.,* **59**, 975–976 (1981)

34. KAY, P. H. and PANETH, M. Aortic valve replacement in the over seventy age group. *J. Cardiovasc Surg.,* **22**, 312–315 (1981)

35. SUKKAR, A. Z., COOPAR, D. K. C., DeNOBREGA, J. *et al.* Valve replacement in patients over 70 years of age. *S. Afr. Med. J.,* **65**, 370–373 (1984)

36. JAMIESON, W. R. E., THOMPSON, D. M. and MUNRO, A. I. Cardiac valve replacement in elderly patients. *Can. Med. Assoc. J.,* **123**, 628–632 (1980)

37. BERGDAHL, L., BJORK, V. O. and JONASSON, R. Aortic valve replacement in patients over 70 years. *Scand. J. Thorac. Cardiovasc. Surg.,* **15**, 123–128 (1981)

38. AROM, K. V., NICOLOFF, D. M., LINDSAY, W. G. *et al.* Should valve replacement and related procedures be performed in elderly patients? *Ann. Thorac. Surg.,* **38**, 466–470 (1984)

39. NICOLAOU, N. and KINSLEY, R. H. Mitral valve replacement in the elderly. *S. Afr. Med. J.*, **65**, 598–600 (1984)

40. HOCKBERG, M. S., DERKAC, W. M., CONKLE, D. M. *et al.* Mitral valve replacement in elderly patients: encouraging postoperative clinical and hemodynamic results. *J. Thorac. Cardiovasc. Surg.*, **77**, 422–426 (1979)

41. CRAVER, J. M., GOLDSTEIN, J., JONES, E. L. *et al.* Clinical, hemodynamic and operative descriptors affecting outcome of aortic valve replacement in elderly vs young patients. *Ann. Surg.*, **199**, 733–741 (1984)

42. MOCK, M. B., HOLMES, D. R., VLIETSTRA, R. E. *et al.* Percutaneous transluminal coronary angioplasty (PTCA) in the elderly patient: experience in the National Heart, Lung, and Blood Institute PTCA Registry. *Am. J. Cardiol.*, **53**, 89c–91c (1984)

43. DORROS, G., COWLEY, M. J., JANKE, L. *et al.* In-hospital mortality rate in the National Heart, Lung and Blood Institute Percutaneous Transluminal Coronary Angioplasty Registry. *Am. J. Cardiol.*, **53**, 17c–21c (1984)

44. DETRE, K. M., MYLER, R. K., KELSEY, S. F. *et al.* Baseline characteristics of patients in the National Heart, Lung and Blood Institute Percutaneous Transluminal Coronary Angioplasty Registry. *Am. J. Cardiol.*, **53**, 7c–11c (1984)

45. JONES, E. L., ABI-MANSOUR, P. and GRUNTZIG, A. R. Coronary artery bypass surgery and percutaneous transluminal coronary angioplasty in the elderly patient. *Cardiology*, **73**, 223–234 (1986)

46. McCALLISTER, B. D., HARTZLER, G. O., REED, W. A. and JOHNSON, T. W. Percutaneous transluminal coronary angioplasty in the elderly: a comparison with coronary bypass surgery. *J. Am. Coll. Cardiol.*, **1**, 656 (1983)

47. TAYLOR, G. J., RABINOVICH, E., MIKELL, F. C. *et al.* Percutaneous transluminal coronary angioplasty: a palliation for patients considered poor surgical candidates. *Am. Heart J.*, **111**, 840–844 (1986)

48. CRIBIER, A., SAOUDI, N., BERLAND, J. *et al.* Percutaneous transluminal balloon valvuloplasty of acquired aortic stenosis in elderly patients: an alternative to valve replacement? *Lancet*, **1**, 63–67 (1986)

49. McKAY, R. G., SAFIAN, R. D. and LOCK, J. E. Balloon dilatation of calcific aortic stenosis in elderly patients: postmortem, intraoperative and percutaneous valvuloplasty studies. *Circulation*, **74**, 119–125 (1986)

50. JACKSON, G., THOMAS, S., MONAGHAN, M. *et al.* Inoperable aortic stenosis in the elderly: benefit from percutaneous transluminal valvuloplasty. *Br. Med. J.*, **294**, 83–86 (1987)

51. REYNOLDS, D. J. M., STONE, D. L., WELLS, F. C. and PETCH, M. C. How does aortic balloon valvuloplasty work? *Br. Heart J.*, **57**, 70 (1987)

Chapter 5

Non-Parkinsonian movement disorders in the elderly

J. R. Playfer

Movement disorders other than Parkinson's disease have been a neglected subject in geriatric literature. This is surprising as some of the most important of these disorders are seen most commonly in the elderly[1]. Tardive dyskinesia and benign essential tremor give rise to unresolved problems in management[2]. A number of the other causes of abnormal involuntary movements such as chorea, athetosis, myoclonus, torsion dystonia, tics and de la Tourette movements, are in general more common in the young and have been the focus of considerable neurophysiological and neurological research in recent years, but, increasingly, examples of these conditions are recognized in the elderly even though their origins may have been in childhood or young adulthood. Some knowledge of these disorders is necessary to sort out the difficult differential diagnoses which these conditions can present to the clinician. While this review concentrates on tardive dyskinesia and tremor, it will also attempt to give an overview of other disorders and to give some idea of the neuroanatomical and neurophysiological basis of these disorders.

By convention, movement disorders usually refer to those conditions that arise from pathology in the basal ganglia so that I will not be discussing cerebellar disorders. Most areas of the cerebral cortex project a sensory input into the corpus striatum of the basal ganglia (see Figure 5.1). These inputs are topographically specific and in the main excitatory in nature, the principal

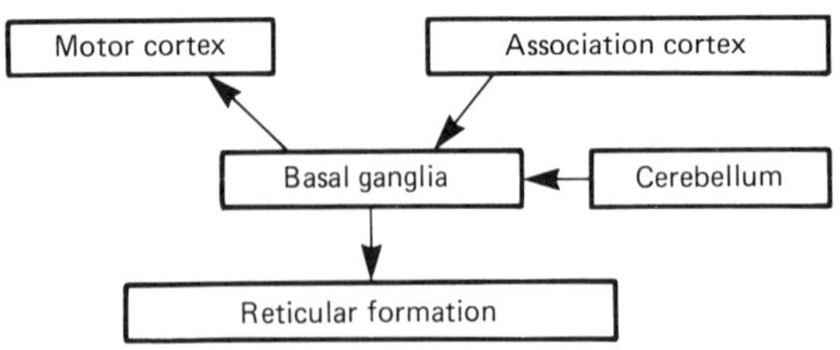

Figure 5.1 Main functional connections of the basal ganglia

neurotransmitter being glutamate. In addition, the corpus striatum receives inputs from the thalamus, particularly the intralamellar nuclei. Although these are also excitatory they are not topographically precise, the neurotransmitters acting as local hormones. The information from this input ultimately projects to the globus pallidus, the output of which is inhibitory, to the reticular formation and the anterior and ventral nuclei of the thalamus. From these nuclei, which also contain inputs from the cerebellum, projections occur to the motor and pre-motor cortex. It can be seen that a crude feedback loop occurs, with excitatory impulses from the cortex, projected to the basal ganglia, resulting in an output of the thalamus, relaying to the motor cortex. The substantia nigra of the basal ganglia is linked to other parts of the basal ganglia with reciprocal connections, particularly with the corpus striatum and the globus pallidus. The substantia nigra also projects downwards to the brainstem reticular formation. The pathways linking the substantia nigra with the corpus striatum employ Substance P as their excitatory transmitter and GABA as their inhibitory transmitter. The reciprocal pathway from the substantia nigra to the corpus striatum employs dopamine as its main transmitter. This appears to have both inhibitory and excitatory functions[3].

Damage to this complex system engenders a bewildering variety of movement disorders. The consequences of neurological damage may result in either deficiency syndromes such as the bradykinesia of Parkinson's disease or release phenomena such as the abnormal involuntary movements which we are to discuss. Curious and often complex movement disorders are observed in elderly people which may be unique, reflecting neuroanatomical or neurophysiological changes which may give indications to basic sciences about the organization of these systems. Basal ganglia can be seen as the source of the basic patterns of movement like a central store of computer programs which are activated by sensory cues received from the cortex. These basic movements are refined by the motor cortex and the cerebellum into organized voluntary movements. When this process is disrupted by pathology crude prototype movements emerge. These give rise to the familiar patterns of chorea, athetosis, balismus, along with the dystonias, tics, tremors etc.

While Parkinson's disease is not the topic of this chapter, it is of course the major movement disorder of geriatric medicine and it is important therefore, before dealing with more specific disorders, to clear the ground as to the number of akinetic-rigid syndromes which may be mistaken for Parkinson's disease (see Table 5.1).

Table 5.1 Akinetic–rigid syndromes

Arteriosclerotic pseudo-Parkinsonism
Normal pressure hydrocephalus
Steele–Richardson–Olszewski syndrome
Shy–Drager syndrome
Alzheimer's disease

Some of these are extremely rare but important because remedial treatment is available. Others are extremely common and important only in so much as there is a poor expectation of response to anti-Parkinsonian drugs. Arteriosclerotic pseudo-Parkinsonism as described by Macdonald Critchley is a familiar pattern seen by geriatricians[4]. This condition has a stepwise progression, associated with cognitive loss. Typically the patient has a 'magnetic' gait and also associated upper motor neurone signs. The pathology of the brain shows small punctate lacunae, presumably due to small infarcts. The condition has a worse prognosis than idiopathic Parkinson's disease and there is little or no response to levodopa. Normal pressure hydrocephalus is a rare condition but is important to recognize[5]. It is characterized by the triad of ataxic gait, incontinence with indifference and mental confusion. About half the cases have a previous history of head injury, meningitis or subarachnoid haemorrhage. Shunting using a Spitz–Holter valve or a similar device can be very effective in relieving symptoms, but in many patients who are elderly there is also cerebral atrophy and these patients do not derive as much benefit from shunting. Steele–Richardson–Olszewski syndrome or supranuclear palsy is a condition with marked axial rigidity, particularly associated with falls and retropulsion[6]. Upper motor neurone signs are usually present. There is a failure of upward gaze, and, later, gaze in other directions, indicating supranuclear involvement of the cranial nerves concerned with eye movement. This syndrome once again has a very poor prognosis and does not respond to levodopa. Shy–Drager syndrome is an example of a variety of disorders classified as multiple system atrophy. It is a disorder primarily of the autonomic nervous system; it presents predominantly with the effects of postural hypotension, often associated with urinary incontinence and impotence. The postural hypotension is the most obvious feature and causes great disability, there may also be extrapyramidal and cerebellar signs. It is a very rare condition, and usually presents in middle life[7]. Alzheimer's disease may frequently be confused or indeed overlap with Parkinson's disease in elderly patients. Advanced cases give rise to severe akinetic rigid phenomena and marked alterations in tone and abnormalities of movement[8]. These features of dementia have been highlighted in the past by the work of George Adams[9]. Usually the dementia is the most marked feature and there are often associated extrapyramidal signs. There is a poor response to levodopa[10].

Choreiform movements form a major group of disorders. Movements of this type are a feature of tardive dyskinesia (see Table 5.2). They are defined as irregular and twitching movements. They occur at random, although they appear to flow from

Table 5.2 Chorea

Associated with neuropathology
  1 Striatal pathology
    Huntington's chorea
    Senile chorea

  2 Diffuse pathology
    Sydenham's chorea
    Systemic lupus erythematosus

Without known cerebral pathology
  Hyperthyroidism
  Hepatocellular syndromes
  Pregnancy
  Drug-induced causes

---

one part of the body to another and thus give the appearance of having a rhythmical element. Gait is highly abnormal, stuttering and halting, and balance is impaired. Chorea may occur as a result of lesions in the striatum. This is typically so in Huntington's chorea and senile chorea. It also arises from diffuse disorders of the brain as in Sydenham's chorea and systemic lupus erythematosus (SLE). A number of conditions give rise to chorea without any known cerebral pathology – hyperthyroidism, hepato-cellular dysfunction and even pregnancy. By far the commonest cause of chorea is drug treatment resulting in tardive dyskinesia. Huntington's chorea and senile chorea need some clarification. Huntington's chorea is a disorder which is most often seen in young adults and middle age[11]. There are exceptional cases which are described in the literature where true Huntington's chorea presents over the age of 60[12]. The dominant gene responsible for Huntington's chorea is located on the short arm of chromosome 4 and is linked to the G8 gene which can be readily identified using

DNA recombination technology[13]. Within individual families, inheritance studies can now determine the risks of offspring being affected by the disease. Compared with Huntington's chorea, senile chorea is a much less well-defined condition in which there is loss of cells in the putamen and caudate nucleus, which is often associated with other neurological damage such as Alzheimer's disease or multi-infarct cerebrovascular disease. It represents possibly an example of accelerated ageing with the brunt of the damage falling on the corpus striatum[14].

Choreiform movements are often associated with, and difficult to distinguish from, athetosis which comprises more sinuous involuntary movements, not as jerky as the movements of chorea[15]. Movements are a delicate alteration between flexion and hyperextension at the wrists and other joints. Unlike chorea, there is some repetition within movements. These movements are associated with a variety of pathology in the basal ganglia, most of which refer to childhood illnesses such as birth injury and metabolic disorders. In the elderly the movements are generally only seen in association with tardive dyskinesia or levodopa-induced dyskinesias. Even more bizarre than chorea or athetosis are ballismic movements, which are sudden movements of the limbs. The limbs project outwards, with considerable force, sometimes engendering serious injuries such as fractures[16]. Ballismic movements are usually confined to one side of the body (hemiballismus) and occur sporadically in old people, the most common pathology being cerebrovascular disease, involving the contralateral subthalamic nucleus. These movements often occur about 4–5 weeks after a cerebrovascular accident. They are worse in the initial phases and often subside over a period of 2–3 months. One can give a reasonably good prognosis if they are not associated with other neurological damage.

The treatment of the three related movement disorders – chorea, athetosis and ballismus – is very difficult and it is only in chorea that we can successfully modify the symptoms. Chorea neuropharmacologically results from enhanced dopaminergic activity, relative to the antagonistic cholinergic and possibly gabanergic systems. Enhanced dopaminergic activity may result from increased concentrations of dopamine presynaptically, or failure to detoxify dopamine or changes in either quantity or quality of dopamine receptors. Intensive treatment by modifying these factors has met with varying success. The mainstay of treatment has been the use of dopamine antagonists such as tetrabenazine. In addition, drugs such as haloperidol have also been found to be useful. Cholinergic agonists such as physostigmine have been tried, particularly in Huntington's chorea, but the short action of the drug has limited its value. Modification of the gabanergic system with drugs such as sodium valproate has been tried with varying success.

The most common movement disorder seen in the elderly is tardive dyskinesia, which results from the long-term action of the neuroleptic drugs, phenothiazines and butyrophenones[17]. The incidence of these reactions increases with age. Neuroleptic drugs are known as such because they can induce Parkinsonism by means of blocking dopamine receptors. This property is associated with a wide range of neurological side-effects. The earliest problem which may arise is an acute dystonic reaction, usually presenting as an oculogyric crisis. These acute problems are more common in younger patients[18]. The generalized motor restlessness akathisia (from the Greek meaning 'restless feet') is often seen in the earlier stages of treatment[19]. This phenomenon is most frequently seen on psychiatric wards and is particularly likely to affect older patients; aimless motor restlessness and repetitive fidgeting characterize the disorder. In contrast, tardive dyskinesia is, as the name implies, late in onset, and usually only develops after many months of treatment. Most typically, tardive dyskinesia comprises abnormal involuntary movements involving the mouth, tongue and facial muscles – the so-called orobucco-facial dyskinesias. Abnormal movements of the trunk and limbs are more commonly seen in the closely related levodopa-induced dyskinesias. Although respiration, speech and feeding can be disrupted by these movements, they are, on the whole, remarkably well tolerated. Tardive dyskinesia shortens life expectancy, the most likely reasons being an increased incidence of bronchopneumonia due to inhalation, and nutritional disorders[20]. The abnormal movements are abolished during sleep and are made worse by activity and emotional arousal. Occasional patients with dyskinesias who have no previous history of exposure to phenothiazines or butyrophenones are seen and presumably suffer from non-specific neurological degeneration. However, it is almost impossible to exclude previous exposure to drugs and these abnormal movements may arise many months after stopping a neuroleptic drug[21]. A curious phenomenon in this condition is that stopping the offending drug usually leads to an exacerbation of the abnormal movements[22]. About one-fifth of patients taking drugs that cause tardive dyskinesia will develop the condition if they are on the drugs for more than a year, and in over half of these patients the dyskinesias will persist after stopping the drug[23]. The older the patient, the greater the risk of developing these movements, and surveys of old people's homes and long-stay psychiatric wards have shown a prevalence of up to 30% amongst patients over the age of 70[24].

The differential diagnosis of tardive dyskinesia is somewhat curious – not many differential diagnoses can contain ill-fitting dentures (Table 5.3). It is, however, important to exclude Huntington's chorea or senile chorea and it is also important to consider drugs such as metoclopramide and prochlorperazine which also have dopamine-blocking activity and may cause the condition[25].

Table 5.3 Differential diagnosis of tardive dyskinesia

Ill-fitting dentures
Senile orofacial dyskinesia
Levadopa dyskinesia
Huntington's chorea
Senile chorea

There is a large literature concerned with the pathophysiology and treatment of tardive dyskinesia[26]. Because of its obvious relationship to Huntington's chorea and levodopa-induced dyskinesia, it seems probable that this condition is due to excessive or abnormal dopaminergic activity. There are several hypotheses as to why the condition should occur. The most probable is that of dopamine receptor supersensitivity. It is considered that when dopamine receptors are blocked, postsynaptic cells produce more dopamine receptors which exhibit 'denervation sensitivity'. There are many problems with this model and other workers have stressed the importance of the compensatory changes that occur in other neurotransmitters once dopamine is blocked, particularly affecting acetylcholine and GABA. There are a number of animal models, rodents being extensively used. Experiments with these models indicate that blocking of the D2 dopamine receptor is more important than the D1 receptor and this opens the door to more specific neuroleptics which do not bind with the D2 receptor. Although there is no pure drug of this sort available at present, sulpiride does not cause tardive dyskinesia and can be used in some psychotic conditions, but is not very effective[26].

For most side-effects, the obvious step is to withdraw the offending drug. In tardive dyskinesia this usually causes an exacerbation of the condition. This may be due to the release of dopamine receptors, causing greater supersensitivity effects. In many conditions in which neuroleptics are used it is impossible to withdraw the drug and certainly in chronic schizophrenia it is preferable to have abnormal movements than frank psychotic behaviour. In the elderly these drugs must be used with great caution and only where there is a clear indication for their use. Where neuroleptics cannot be stopped without causing major difficulties, there is a range of therapeutic options which may be tried. As is so often the case, a wide range of drugs available indicates that none is ideal, and often drug treatment of tardive dyskinesia is depressingly ineffective. The most common approach is to use anti-dopaminergic drugs. These can be classified into two types – dopamine blockers and dopamine depletors. Tetrabenazine is an agent which combines both of these actions and is probably the most widely used drug in this condition[27]. In longer-term use, it exhibits reserpine-like qualities causing over-sedation and depression. It is an extremely difficult drug to use in the elderly, although it is effective in suppressing some abnormal movements.

The ergot alkaloid compound co-dergocrine mesylate (Hydergine) is an interesting compound which has some theoretical advantages in the treatment of tardive dyskinesia. It is a partial dopamine agonist, having dopaminergic activity at very low concentrations of dopamine and becoming a dopamine antagonist as the levels of dopamine rise. Thus in theory this drug could be used as a switch. When dopamine is depleted it has some agonist action, avoiding the complete sedative effects of the dopamine depletors. On the other hand, when dopamine activity is in excess, causing abnormal movements, it can switch off the action of dopamine. In a series of studies using an intravenous challenge technique this drug is able to reduce the number of involuntary movements[28]. Its use as an oral agent, however, is extremely difficult and though double-blind controlled trials have shown that it does reduce abnormal involuntary movements when taken orally, there are some curious features, such as the fact that the tardive dyskinesia continues to improve after stopping the drug[29]. Unfortunately this drug has not as yet found a place in this condition, although it could yet prove an effective agent.

Small doses of dopamine agonists such as bromocriptine and apomorphine, used in order to stimulate the presynaptic dopamine receptor, thus switching off the endogenous synthesis and release of dopamine, have been tried with some success, but the dosage is critical and if incorrect can greatly exacerbate the condition[30]. The use of cholinergic drugs or pro-drugs, such as choline and lecithin, in an effort to increase cholinergic activity to balance the excessive dopaminergic activity, was shown to be of little use in tardive dyskinesia[31,32]. Drugs that modify GABA activity, such as sodium valproate, baclofen or benzodiazepines, still have their advocates for this condition although well designed, good, double-blind controlled studies have failed to show major benefit[33–35]. The side-effects, particularly hypotonia, dizziness, confusion and drowsiness, are common at the high doses needed to modify abnormal movements. Propanolol is another agent that has been tried and some success claimed; however these claims are doubtful[36].

Prevention is always the best form of medicine and there is no doubt that the restriction and careful use of neuroleptic drugs would greatly reduce the prevalence of tardive dyskinesia. The practice of giving anti-cholinergic drugs as a routine to patients on antipsychotic drugs has now been shown to increase the incidence of abnormal involuntary movements and does nothing to prevent Parkinsonism[37]. As noted earlier, the commonly used drugs metoclopramide and prochlorperazine have dopa-blocking activity and have been implicated in the production of drug-induced Parkinson's disease and abnormal movements[38]. Domperidone would seem a much safer alternative as this drug does not penetrate the blood–brain barrier to the same extent.

The diagnosis of tremor in an elderly patient can be extremely difficult. The most commonly occurring tremor is what was formerly called benign essential tremor; it is now more generally known as idiopathic tremor. This condition was described in detail by Macdonald Critchley in 1949[39], and extensively reviewed by Lee in 1987[40]. Idiopathic tremor differs from Parkinsonian tremor, being largely an action tremor in contrast to the resting tremor of Parkinson's disease. It also has a slightly higher frequency of 8–10 cycles per second. The condition has a positive family history in 50% of patients. There have been claims that it is a simple autosomal dominant characterized by a late expression of the gene, but it is unusual for a simple genetic disorder to express itself in late middle age and old age. It affects predominantly the hands when they are being used in holding a cup, fastening clothes etc. The amplitude of the tremor is variable, but noticeably affects such activities as handwriting and feeding. The tremor has to be distinguished from an intention tremor, and also from tremors produced by drugs such as salbutamol, phenytoin or sodium valproate. It is a well-known clinical fact that about 50% of these tremors can improve on taking alcohol[41]. Some authorities have claimed that primidone is a useful drug, although risks of side-effects are high in the elderly[42]. Propranolol is helpful in some cases, particularly those with rapid fine tremor[43].

There are a large number of disorders which are neurological curios in the elderly and are mainly seen in younger patients; some are extremely rare even within that group. Dystonic conditions, particularly torsion dystonia, are more common in younger individuals. They are disorders of the co-activation of different muscle groups, affecting limbs, trunk, head and neck, causing the body to be pulled into often bizarre and painful postures. Although considered a disorder of the basal ganglia, there are no gross pathological changes there. These disorders may arise in relation to infection or cerebral infarction. In some instances drugs may be implicated, in particular levodopa. Patients who have suffered from lifelong cerebral palsy present with dystonic features in old age[44]. Clonazepam and carbamazepine have been tried with some success in this condition[45]. Focal dystonias such as torticollis and writer's cramp may present in any age, including old age[46].

Myoclonus is a condition which has attracted considerable attention from neurophysiologists and neurologists in recent years[47]. Myoclonus is a sudden, non-rhythmical contraction which may be focal, involving one muscle or a small group of muscles, or it may be generalized, resembling a startle response. Myoclonus may be caused by a large number of factors, some of which are relatively common conditions in the elderly, most notably Alzheimer's or Jakob–Creuzfeldt disease and progressive supranuclear palsy. Tics and habit spasms almost exclusively develop before old age, yet once established may persist throughout life. Movements are brief, purposeless and repetitive. There is usually some ability to suppress them, but once they are well established this diminishes. They vary from very simple movements to extremely complicated ones as seen in Gilles de la Tourette syndrome[48]. One particular form which is noteworthy in geriatric medicine is blepharospasm – involuntary forceful and sustained closure of the eyelids. This was a notable feature in patients with post-encephalitic Parkinsonism, but is also seen in patients with advanced dementia and in patients with levodopa-induced dyskinesia[49].

References

1. DALZIEL, J. A. *Geriat. Med.*, **12,** November, 25–28 (1982)
2. JESTE, D. W. and WYAT, R. J. *Understanding and Treating Tardive Dyskinesias*, Guilford Press, New York (1982)
3. STEIN, J. F. *An Introduction to Neurophysiology*, Blackwell Scientific, Oxford, pp. 271–280 (1982)

4. CRITCHLEY, M. In *Research Progress in Parkinson's Disease* (ed. F. Clifford Rose and R. Capildeo), Pitman, London, pp. 40–43 (1981)
5. LEES, A. J. *Med. Int.*, **1**, 32 (1983)
6. MAHER, E. R. and LEES, A. J. *Neurology*, **36**, 1005–1008 (1986)
7. SPOKES, E. G., BANNISTER, R., OPPENHEIMER, D. R. *J. Neurol. Sci.*, **43**, 59–82 (1979)
8. PAULSON, G. W. In *Dementia*, 2nd edn (ed. C. E. Wells), F. A. Davies, Philadelphia (1977)
9. ADAMS, G. *Br. Med. J.*, **3**, 789–791 (1976)
10. TURNBULL, C. J. and AITKEN, J. A. *Age Ageing*, **12**, 309 (1983)
11. MARSDEN, C. D. In *Textbook of Medicine* (ed. D. J. Weatherall, J. G. G. Ledingham and D. Warrell), Oxford Medical Publications, Oxford, pp. 21–113 (1983)
12. MYERS, R. H., SAX, D. S., SHOERFIELD, M. and BIRD, E. D. *J. Neurol. Neurosurg. Psychiat.*, **48**, 530–534 (1985)
13. GUSELLA, J. F., TANZI, R. E., ANDERSON, M. A. *et al. Science*, **225**, 2829–2833 (1984)
14. BRUYN, G. W. *Huntington's Chorea. Handbook of Clinical Neurology*, vol. 6, North Holland, Amsterdam, pp. 298–377 (1968)
15. CARPENTER, M. B. *Arch. Neurol. Psychiat.*, **63**, 875 (1950)
16. LEES, A. J. *Med. Int.*, **32**, 1516 (1983)
17. MARSDEN, C. D. and FAHN, S. In *Movement Disorders 2* (ed. C. D. Marsden and S. Fahn), Butterworth Scientific, Guildford, pp. 305–313 (1987)
18. WEINER, W. J. and KLAWSON, H. C. *J. Am. Geriat. Soc.*, **21**, 318–320 (1973)
19. MARSDEN, C. D. and FAHN, S. In *Movement Disorders* (ed. C. D. Marsden and S. Fahn), Butterworth Scientific, Guildford, ch. 12, pp. 192–193 (1982)
20. PAULSON, G. W. In *Disorders of Movement* (ed. A. Barbeau), MTP Press, Lancaster, ch. 7, pp. 133–151 (1981)
21. MARSDEN, C. D., MINDHAM, R. H. S. and MACKAY, A. V. P. In *The Pharmacology and Treatment of Schizophrenia* (ed. P. B. Bradley and S. R. Hirsch), Oxford University Press, Oxford (1983)
22. QUITKIN, F., RIFKIN, A., GAUFIELD, L. and KLEIN, D. F. *Am. J. Psychol.*, **135**, 371 (1977)
23. VILLENEUVE, A. and BOGORNERGI, Z. *Lancet*, **1**, 353 (1970)
24. BLOWER, A. Tardive dyskinesia in old people's homes. *Proceedings of the British Geriatrics Society*, Liverpool (1983)
25. ORME, M. and TALLIS, R. C. *Br. Med. J.*, **289**, 397–398 (1984)
26. ANON. *Drug. Ther. Bull.*, **24**, 7 (1986)
27. MACALLUM, W. A. *Br. Med. J.*, **1**, 760 (1970)
28. PLAYFER, J. R., GAUTUM, P., SNAPE, J. *et al. Proceedings of the British Geriatric Society*, Dublin (1984)
29. HAJIOFF, J. and WALLACE, M. *Psycho. Pharmacol.*, **79**, 1–3 (1983)
30. JESTE, D. V., CUTLER, N. R., KAUFMAN, C. A. and KAROOM, F. *Biol. Psychiat.*, **18**, 1085–1091 (1983)
31. GROWDON, J. M., HIRSCH, M. J., WURTMAN, R. J. and WIENER, W. *N. Engl. J. Med.*, **297**, 524 (1977)
32. GOETZ, C. G., WEINER, W. J. and KLAWANS, H. L. In *Disorders of Movement* (ed. A. Barbeau), MTP Press, Lancaster, pp. 29–37 (1981)
33. PRICE, P. A., PARKES, J. D. and MARSDEN, C. D. *J. Neurol. Neurosurg. Psychiat.*, **41**, 702 (1978)
34. KORSGAARO, S. *Acta Psychiat. Scand.*, **54**, 17 (1976)
35. PEIRIS, J. B., BORALESSA, H. and LICREL, N. P. W. *Med. J. Aust.*, **1**, 225 (1976)
36. RISCH, S. C., COHEN, R. M. and KALIN, N. H. *Am. J. Psychiat.*, **137**, 1125 (1980)
37. GARDOS, G. and COLE, J. O. *Am. J. Psychiat.*, **135**, 1321–1324 (1983)

38. DAVIS, W. A. *N. Engl. J. Med.*, **294**, 113 (1976)
39. CRITCHLEY, M. *Brain*, **72**, 113–139 (1949)
40. LEE, R. G. In *Movement Disorders 2* (ed. C. D. Marsden and S. Fahn), Butterworth Scientific, Guildford, pp. 423–438 (1987)
41. GROWDON, J. H., SHAHANI, B. T., YOUNG, R. R. *Neurology*, **25**, 259 (1975)
42. FINDLEY, M. and McLELLAN, D. L. *Br. Med. J.*, **285**, 808 (1985)
43. WILKINSON, P. R., DIXON, N. and HUNTER, K. R. *J. Int. Res.*, **2**, 220 (1974)
44. ROTHWELL, J. C. and OBESO, J. H.. In *Movement Disorders 2* (ed. C. D. Marsden and S. Fahn), Butterworth Scientific, Guildford, pp. 313–332 (1987)
45. McLELLAN, D. L. In *The Clinical Neurology of Old Age* (ed. R. C. Tallis), Wiley, London (1988)
46. HUGHES, M. and McLELLAN, D. L. *J. Neurol. Neurosurg. Psychiat.*, **48**, 782–787 (1985)
47. MARSDEN, C. D., HALLET, M. and FAHN, S. In *Movement Disorders* (ed. C. D. Marsden and S. Fahn), Butterworth Scientific, London, ch. 13, pp. 196–248 (1982)
48. FAHN, S. In *Gilles de la Tourette Syndrome* (ed. A. J. Friedhoff and T. N. Chese), *Advances in Neurology,* vol. 35, Raven Press, New York, pp. 341–344 (1982)
49. JON KOVIN, J. and FORD, J. *Ann. Neurol.*, **13**, 402–411 (1983)

Chapter 6

The autonomic nervous system and postural hypotension in the elderly

Michael Lye

The autonomic nervous system has fascinated physiologists for decades. The system has been seen as the homeostatic regulator of the body which, by sensing changes in the internal and external environments and by reacting to these stimuli, returns the system or whole organism back towards some homeostatic set-point. It is only in the more recent past that clinicians involved with patient care have come to appreciate fully the central regulatory role of the autonomic nervous system in illness and in health. The main impetus to this newer interest stems from what may fairly be called an explosion in pharmacological knowledge, in particular, appreciation of receptor functions and the development of potent receptor agonists and antagonists.

A further stimulus to the renewed interest in the autonomic nervous system has been provided by the recognition that the system is intimately involved with, and acts in concert with, the endocrine system. The complex inter-reactions of the sympathetic component of the autonomic nervous system and the renin-angiotensin-aldosterone hormonal orchestra have opened new therapeutic avenues, particularly in the field of cardiovascular homeostasis. The age of 'designer drugs' suggests even more exciting possibilities in these areas within the next few years.

The expansion of recent information about the autonomic nervous system has wrested study of the system from the neurologists, with their emphasis on nosological classification and their anatomical obsessions, to cardiologists, respirologists and pharmacologists who are more interested in the dynamics of the system and how its responses may be manipulated. With one or two exceptions, gerontologists and geriatricians have, apart from the isolated syndrome of hypothermia, shown less interest in the autonomic nervous system. This is both a surprise and perhaps a wasted opportunity. It is anticipated that this position will change in the future and will yield even more exciting possibilities in the areas of normal ageing and age-related diseases.

A characteristic of the biological ageing process is that it renders the organism less able to respond to phenomena that perturb a homeostatic equilibrium. An aged organism does not appreciate disturbances in equilibrium as quickly as does a younger one, allows more deviation from set-point and, finally, reacts slower and less efficiently to restore normality. It is inconceivable that the autonomic nervous system and neuroendocrine systems are not involved in this ageing phenomenon. Unfortunately, little research has been applied and our knowledge of the impact of ageing on these systems is, as yet, embryonic.

Organization of the autonomic nervous system

Morphologically, the autonomic nervous system consists of two major components – the adrenergic sympathetic and the cholinergic parasympathetic arms. Classically it was thought that the two arms acted like a see-saw – one being excitatory to an end organ with the other acting as an inhibitor[1]. This simple 'checks and balances' system has had to be modified as more and more subdivisions have been uncovered[2,3]. The complex outlined in Figure 6.1 no doubt will itself be elaborated and modified in the near future.

It is important to appreciate that the outline (Figure 6.1) of receptors does not represent a fixed entity. Receptors themselves are dynamic and can up-regulate or down-regulate depending upon the prevailing tone of the system. Equally, the activity of both receptors and of the various relay stations within the

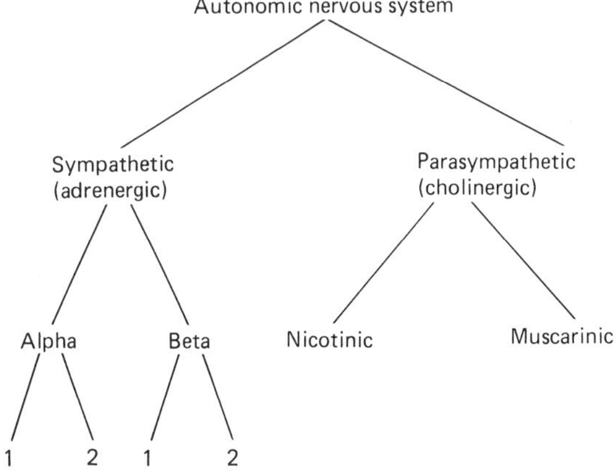

Figure 6.1 Organization of the autonomic nervous system

autonomic nervous system are subject to modulation by the endocrine system (renin–angiotensin–aldosterone) and vasopressin. Finally, activity of the autonomic nervous system is considerably altered by therapeutic agents. Obviously the various direct and specific receptor agonists and antagonists produce (usually!) predictable results. Others may not. For example, non-steroidal anti-inflammatory agents via their prostaglandin synthetase inhibitory action markedly change juxtaglomerular release of renin producing 'knock-on' effects within the autonomic nervous system.

Function of the autonomic nervous system

Alpha-adrenoceptors are mainly located within the peripheral vascular tree whilst the beta-adrenergic system innervates the heart and gastrointestinal tract, though there is some functional overlap. Increase in alpha-1 adrenoceptor activity leads to peripheral (skin) vasoconstriction, pupillary mydriasis and, to a lesser extent, intestinal relaxation and hepatic glycogenolysis. Alpha-2 activity decreases lipolysis and reduces renin output by the juxtaglomerular apparatus.

Beta-1 adrenoceptors are confined to the heart. Increased beta-1 tone increases cardiac contractility (positive inotropism), increases heart rate (positive chronotropism) and decreases the refractory period. Beta-2 adrenoceptors are much more widely distributed. Those located within muscles cause vasodilatation and increase blood flow, especially during exercise. Their actions within the respiratory system (bronchodilatation) have been well exploited using specific beta-2 agonists in the treatment of asthma. Within the gastrointestinal tract increased beta-2 activity leads to intestinal dilatation and increased glycogenolysis. Finally, beta-2 receptors play an important role in uterine relaxation during parturition, when activity is potentiated by other changes in the hormonal background.

The differentiation in functional terms between muscarinic and nicotinic parasympathetic cholinergic activity is not as clear as with the adrenergic subsets. Increased parasympathetic tone acts in the opposite way to increased beta-1 adrenergic activity on the heart and bronchi. Intestinal, ureteric and bladder motility is increased. Miosis occurs and there is increased secretion from the lachrymal and salivary glands. Increased exocrine sweat secretion is primarily a muscarinic effect of parasympathetic activity, as are effects of receptors involving some peripheral blood vessels.

Effects of ageing

With increasing age in healthy humans there are increasing histological signs of segmental Schwann-cell disruption and breakages within the myelin sheaths of autonomic fibres. Direct measurement of nervous transmission through autonomic ganglia and nerve conduction velocity demonstrates an almost linear decline with increasing age beyond puberty. These age-associated electrical changes correspond to the histological findings. Unfortunately the presence of arteriosclerosis inducing pathological lesions of neurones and their processes has not been adequately excluded[4]. That said, it does however remain highly probable that ageing *per se* does impair autonomic function[5]. The extent of impairment remains unquantified.

Many studies of receptor function in relation to increasing age have been carried out over the years. The dose of phenylephrine needed to elevate blood pressure increases with increasing age of subject, suggesting an age-effect on alpha-1 adrenoceptor function. Noradrenaline-induced aortic contractility involving alpha-2 adrenoceptors also declines with increasing age. However, many studies have not taken into acount the almost ubiquitous presence of arteriosclerosis in elderly subjects. Mechanical changes in end organs may be more important than the changes in receptors[4]. Studies of human platelet alpha-2 adrenoceptors have yielded inconsistent results. Overall it must be concluded that ageing may reduce peripheral alpha-adrenoceptor responsiveness in man, but the change is of little physiological importance[6].

Beta-adrenoceptor responsiveness declines with increasing age in a more predictable manner than alpha-adrenoceptor responsiveness. This conclusion is based on studies using specific beta-adrenoceptor agonists and antagonists, but again the problem of impaired end organ function (mechanical) is ever present. These studies do not rule out the possibility of age-related impairment of function beyond the level of membrane receptors (see below). Studies of the number of adrenoceptors and the effects of age have been conflicting. Some workers have found significant and reproducible decreases in number with increasing age. Others, using seemingly identical methods and preparations, have found no change in receptors with increasing age. These rather gross differences between studies are not entirely methodological. It is increasingly recognized that the number of receptors of whatever type and in whatever tissue is not fixed but dynamic. They are subject to up- and down-regulation depending upon the ambient tone of the system. Thus if sympathetic tone is high, the system down-regulates and vice versa, and numbers of receptors will change[7].

There is some evidence to suggest that increasing age limits up-regulatory activity without changing down-regulation[8]. The relationship of ligand adrenoceptor affinity and increasing age is unresolved. Some workers find a decrease in affinity with increasing age[9], others find no such relationship. As Docherty and O'Malley[6] have pointed out, however, numbers and affinity of receptors in relation to increasing age may not be an important consideration. Age may affect responsiveness beyond the receptors, i.e. at sub-cellular level; indeed Weiss *et al.*[10] found in rats that the response of cAMP-dependent protein kinase – the final common pathway at subcellular level of adrenergic activity – is attenuated by increasing age. Further work using human tissue is awaited with interest.

The plasma level of noradrenaline represents a small overspill proportion of the neurotransmitter released at postganglionic adrenergic nerve endings. As such, it is a reliable measure of sympathetic activity[11]. Resting plasma noradrenaline increases with increasing age in healthy subjects[12,13]. Further, any stress, physiological or pathological, usually leads to a greater increase of noradrenaline in older subjects[14,15]. This is a real increase and not secondary to an age-related diminished renal clearance[16]. Indeed, the finding that increasing age is associated with increased dopamine beta-hydroxylase activity – a noradrenaline precursor – confirms that basal sympathetic tone is genuinely increased in the elderly[17].

An interesting observation confirmed by Davidson *et al.*[18], is that women have significantly higher levels of plasma noradrenaline than men, and this difference is maintained into old age. This association may suggest that at least some of the age-related rise in plasma levels of the neurotransmitter is due to the age-related increase in proportion of body fat. There is also a relationship between sleep in the elderly and plasma noradrenaline levels[19]. The relationship remains obscure – does raised sympathetic tone impair sleep in the elderly or does broken sleep activate the nervous system? Would adrenergic blocking agents be good and safe physiological hypnotics in the elderly?

Postural hypotension

Physiology

Man has developed upright gait only recently in the course of his evolution. On standing, approximately 500 ml of blood is taken out of the effective circulation by peripheral pooling in dependent parts. The reduced venous return leads to a decrease of more than 30% in stroke volume. The systemic blood pressure drops almost immediately. In order to maintain perfusion pressures for vital organs, a complex reflex involving mainly peripheral vasoconstriction, but also other mechanisms, is initiated. The result is that blood pressure is restored in healthy individuals within 30 s of standing[20]. After this period there is a small, but variable fall in systolic blood pressure and a rise in diastolic pressure, and thus a restoration of pre-standing mean blood pressure levels.

There are a number of interacting regulatory reflexes involved in this process[21]. Aortic and carotid body baroreceptors discharge with the fall in blood pressure and activate the brainstem 'vasomotor centre' leading to an increased adrenergic and a decreased cholinergic output by the autonomic nervous system. Increased sympathetic output increases cardiac contractility and total peripheral resistance whilst parasympathetic withdrawal increases heart rate[22]. Increased sympathetic activity is reflected in a doubling of plasma noradrenaline levels[23].

Other neuroendocrine reflexes affecting cardiovascular homeostasis are perhaps less important in postural regulation as they take longer, minutes to hours, to operate[22]. They include renin–angiotensin, antidiuretic hormone, prostaglandins and aldosterone. However, as discussed earlier, it is highly likely that these hormones modulate, positively or negatively, adrenergic and cholinergic receptor responses and thus alter autonomic nervous system effectiveness. Local 'intrinsic' blood flow changes which redistribute blood flow to vital organs, e.g. brain and heart, are important but ill understood.

Age-associated changes

The effects of age-associated changes in the cardiovascular system on postural regulatory responses have not been studied in detail[24], although isolated individual components have. The afferent (sensory) component of the postural reflex is probably attenuated with increasing age[25], although not all workers would agree. Stroke volume and cardiac output fall *less* on head-up tilt or standing in healthy elderly subjects compared with younger ones[26]. In healthy elderly subjects heart rate increases less, whilst plasma volume changes are similar[26]. Total peripheral resistance increases on head-up tilt less in older subjects, but it is important to note that the supine peripheral resistance is increased with age and therefore the capacity to respond is inevitably attenuated[26].

As already discussed, basal plasma noradrenaline levels are high in older subjects, but the response to tilt is exaggerated[15]. The response of plasma renin activity (PRA), aldosterone and vasopressin to head-up tilt do not change with increasing age, though basal levels of PRA are lower and of vasopressin higher in the elderly[27]. Plasma osmolality levels and changes during tilt are identical in young and old patients, implying that 'leaky veins' are not a consequence of ageing processes[27].

It is difficult to summarize the overall effects of ageing on postural adaptation as no publication is available as yet which reports a study of the haemodynamic and neuroendocrine responses in an integrated fashion in carefully selected elderly subjects[24]. It does seem, however, that with age the qualitative response to posture change is not altered, but the quantitative haemodynamic responses are markedly attenuated. This, taken in conjunction with the enhanced neuroendocrine drive, suggests that any age-associated limitations of homeostatic mechanisms involve primarily peripheral end organs rather than control reflexes[22,28].

Diagnosis and aetiology

The inability to maintain blood pressure on the assumption of the upright posture constitutes the syndrome of postural or orthostatic hypotension. The fall in blood pressure is variably associated with symptoms, presumably some people can compensate for a lower perfusion pressure by cerebral autoregulation thus minimizing symptoms. Hypotension, whether symptomatic or not, may occur in old people during or after exercise or following large carbohydrate meals[29]. The relationship of these two conditions to the syndrome of postural hypotension is unsure – they may well represent one end of a spectrum of cardiovascular instability[30].

The incidence of postural hypotension increases with increasing age. Approximately 15% of people between 65 and 75 years of age will demonstrate significant falls in blood pressure on standing. This proportion doubles beyond the age of 75 years. Diagnosis requires a high index of suspicion – the conjunction of symptoms with changes in posture is not always appreciated by the patient. Simple indirect blood pressure measurement before and after standing will confirm the diagnosis[4]. It is important to allow sufficient time (20 min plus) for blood pressure to settle before the patient stands[31]. Blood pressure should then be recorded 2 and 5 min after standing. A fall of 20 mmHg or more in systolic and/or a fall of 10 mmHg or more in diastolic pressure defines the presence of postural hypotension, whether or not there are any symptoms[22].

The causes of postural hypotension in the elderly are legion; the interested reader is referred to two recent reviews[4,30]. Several points in relation to the elderly bear emphasis. The condition is usually a combination of the age-associated factors discussed above and a number of precipitating and potentiating factors. A single aetiology is unlikely in the elderly. If the clinician does find one, he must look for others. Iatrogenic causes (drugs) may account for upwards of half the cases[22]. Immobility, from whatever cause, deconditions cardiovascular reflexes and may uncover previously unrecognized postural symptoms[32]. Dehydration, often secondary to a respiratory infection, is a potent cause of postural hypotension in the elderly[33]. Neurological lesions are often associated with postural hypotension. Focal (stroke) and diffuse cerebrovascular disease may cause severe postural hypotension. The stroke patient who is slumped, almost semi-conscious sitting in a chair, but is alert in bed, should have the blood pressure measured. Laudable early mobilization should not be at the cost of cerebral blood flow. Specific syndromes of autonomic failure occur less frequently in elderly patients than in young or middle-aged individuals[4]. The two varieties of 'idiopathic orthostatic hypotension' – one, multisystem atrophy, with diffuse neurological degeneration[34], the other either solitary neuropathy or combined with Parkinson's disease – are relatively uncommon in old age. They are easily distinguished by differences in plasma noradrenaline levels[4]. Both types may be associated with sphincter problems. Finally, afferent failure, usually due to diabetes, should not be forgotten.

Management

Because the aetiology of postural hypotension in the elderly is multifactorial, it leads to the suggestion that management should also be multiple. Unfortunately, multiple treatment may imply polypharmacy to some doctors with often dire consequences to the patient. Management involves early recognition of the syndrome, assessment of the precipitating, potentiating and complicating factors, appraisal of the environment, full clinical diagnostic work-up, treatment of specific problems and only then, specific drug treatment of the hypotension. The practitioner who starts with anti-hypotensive therapy is doomed to failure.

A high index of suspicion combined with repeated measures of blood pressure under the precise circumstances which precipitate the symptoms in the patient lead to early recognition of the syndrome. It may require the clinician's taking blood pressures in the patient's home, when the patient first awakes, after a meal, after a bath or after exercise. Measurements need to be repeated over several days because of extreme variability in both symptoms and blood pressure[22]. Some patients have falls of 40 mmHg or more in systolic blood pressure and are asymptomatic; other patients are disabled by a fall of 10 mmHg or even less[35,36].

A detailed search for precipitating and potentiating factors with emphasis on drugs being taken by the patient is the next step. All drugs taken by the patient should be scrutinized carefully. 'Over the counter' drugs which the patient may omit to recall in a drug history should not be forgotten. A visit to the patient's home may reveal a veritable cornucopia of drugs, many of which may be quite ancient. Stopping drugs, changing to another variety, changing the time of administration or dose whilst monitoring the symptoms and blood pressure will identify the causative drug. Particular attention should be paid to all anti-hypertensive agents, sedatives of any type, including short-acting hypnotics, anti-depressants, anti-Parkinsonian drugs and muscle relaxants. Whether one considers alcohol a drug or not, its potent vasodilatory capacity can lead to severe postural hypotension. Alcohol abuse is not uncommon in the elderly.

Alteration of the patient's external environment may be much easier than manipulation of his *milieu intérieur*. Provision of a bath-seat may allow a patient to rise in stages from a hot vasodilating bath. Alternatively, a cold shower may be preferred. Rails may assist rising from the toilet and, by preventing a Valsalva manoeuvre, avoid syncope. Patients should be advised to rise from bed in easy stages. Advice to avoid sudden explosive exercise – walk with dignity not speed – may not be heeded, but is worth a try.

The symptoms of postural hypotension may be non-specific, but to the patient they are often devastating and frightening. This fear leads to a vicious circle – lack of confidence leading to immobility and worsening of the postural hypotension. No drugs help with this complication of postural hypotension[4]. A full multi-disciplinary rehabilitation team of nurses and therapists is required. Confidence can only be restored by a combination of encouragement, support and cajolery. Needless to say, the patient's general condition needs to be optimized as any improvement in physical capabilities will help postural hypotension. After full clinical evaluation, routine haematological and biochemical profiles should be obtained[30]. Chest X-ray may reveal an unsuspected bronchial carcinoma. An abnormal routine 12-lead ECG may indicate the need for a stress (tilt or exercise) test. Routine thyroid function tests may uncover atypical thyrotoxicosis. Serum vitamin B12 and blood sugar measurements are indicated in all elderly patients with postural hypotension. More specific investigations will be as indicated by the initial examination, history and the results from baseline tests. Detailed tests of cardiovascular function are not justified as they will not influence management[22]. Tests of cardiovascular function and reflexes in the older patient have been evaluated and the normal range is established. The interested reader is referred to the publications of Clark and Mapstone[37], Hainsworth and Al-Shamma[38], Kaijiser and Sachs[39], Parnati *et al.*[40] and Vargas *et al.*[15].

The full clinical assessment and investigation should have uncovered at least one pathological condition in the elderly patient with postural hypotension. Most often there will be more. It is wise to asume that any such pathology may be causing or potentiating the postural hypotension[4]. They should, as far as possible, all be treated. A general programme of remobilization will increase the physical capacity of the patient, which in itself may lead to amelioration of symptoms if not the hypotension.

Physical methods of treatment are safe, have no serious adverse effects, and are effective[41]. Full-length hosiery, which includes the waist, is simple and cheap and should be the first step in treatment. The fear that hosiery might actually worsen postural hypotension has not been borne out in practice[22]. These garments need to be carefully fitted and the patient may need instruction in their use and care. The elderly patient may be reluctant to use them initially, but should be encouraged to persist. Sleeping with the head of the bed elevated may be remarkably effective in relieving symptoms with little effect on postural blood pressure falls.

Numerous drugs have been tried in the treatment of postural hypotension[4]. They are all variously effective, but limited by adverse effects. Thus the sympathomimetic agents (amphetamines, methylphenidate, tyramine with or without a monoamine oxidase inhibitor) are effective, at least initially, but lead to supine hypertension[42]. Dihydroergotamine, which has a differential effect on veins and arteries, is occasionally effective but as well as producing supine hypertension, may lead to peripheral gangrene[30]. Low bioavailability is another problem[43]. Mineralocorticoids exemplified by fludrocortisone may produce cardiac failure in the elderly and are best avoided.

Prostaglandin synthetase inhibitors, in the form of non-steroidal anti-inflammatory drugs, have been used to counter the vasodilatory effects of endogenous prostaglandins. They also increase sensitivity of peripheral blood vessels to sympathetic activity[44]. Their adverse effects on the gastrointestinal and renal systems may preclude their use in some elderly patients[45]. Dopamine antagonists (metoclopropramide) may counter the salt-wasting effect of excess dopamine following peripheral adrenergic failure[46]. Extrapyramidal side-effects limit usefulness in the elderly[47].

New agents are being constantly tried in the treatment of this difficult syndrome. Direct adrenergic agents (pindolol) have not lasted long. Xamoterol, a beta-adrenergic blocking agent with very high intrinsic sympathomimetic activity, shows promise, but there is little experience as yet[48]. Arginine vasopressin analogues have been advocated[49] but are unlikely to be particularly efficacious in the elderly who already have enhanced arginine vasopressin levels under stress[50].

References

1. MYERSON, A. *JAMA*, **110**, 101 (1938)
2. AHLQUIST, R. P. *Am. J. Physiol.*, **153**, 586 (1948)
3. LANDS, A. M., ARNOLD, A., McAULIFFE, J. P. *et al. Nature*, **214**, 597 (1967)
4. LYE, M. In *The Clinical Neurology of Old Age* (ed. R. C. Tallis), Wiley, Chichester (1988)
5. COLLINS, K. J. In *Autonomic Failure* (ed. R. Bannister), Oxford University Press, Oxford, p. 489 (1983)
6. DOCHERTY, J. R. and O'MALLEY, K. *Clin. Sci.*, **10** (Suppl. 10), 133S (1985)
7. TASCH, M. D. and STOELTING, R. K. In *Geriatric Anaesthesia* (ed. C. R. Stephen and R. A. E. Assaf), Butterworths, Boston, p. 115 (1986)
8. HUI, K. K. P. and CONNOLLY, M. E. *N. Engl. J. Med.*, **304**, 1473 (1981)
9. KRALL, J. F., CONNOLLY, M., WEISHART, R. and TUCK, M. L. *J. Clin. Endocrinol. Metabol.*, **52**, 863 (1981)
10. WEISS, B., GREENBERG, L. and CANTOR, E. *Fed. Proc.*, **38**, 1915 (1979)
11. ROWE, J. W. and TROEN B. R. *Endocrine Rev.*, **1**, 167 (1980)
12. VEITH, R. C., FEATHERSTONE, J. A., LIVARES, O. A. and HALTER, J. B. *J. Gerontol.*, **41**, 319 (1986)
13. ZIEGLER, M. G., LAKE, C. R. and KOPIN, I. J. *Nature*, **261**, 333 (1976)
14. LEHMAN, M. and KEUL, J. *Eur. J. Appl. Physiol. Occup. Physiol.*, **55**, 302 (1986)
15. VARGAS, E., ROTHWELL, C., WEINKOVE, C. and LYE, M. *Gerontol.*, **30**, 253 (1984)
16. HOELDTKE, R. D. and CILMI, K. M. *J. Clin. Endocrinol. Metabol.*, **60**, 479 (1985)
17. BANERJI, T. K., PARKENING, T. A. and COLLINS, T. J. *J. Gerontol.*, **39**, 264 (1984)
18. DAVIDSON, L., VANDONGEN, R., ROUSE, I. L. *et al. Clin. Sci.*, **67**, 347 (1984)
19. PRINZ, P. N., HALTER, J., BENEDETTI, C. and RASKIND, M. *J. Clin. Endocrinol. Metabol.*, **49**, 300 (1979)

20. CURRENS, J. H. *Am. Heart J.,* **35**, 646 (1948)
21. GUYTON, A. C. In *Developments in Cardiovascular Medicine* (ed. C. J. Dickinson and J. Marks), MTP Press, Lancaster, p. 265 (1978)
22. LYE, M. and VARGAS, E. In *Geriatric Heart Disease* (ed. E. L. Coodley), PSG, Littleton, Mass., p. 189 (1985)
23. LAKE, C. R., ZIEGLER, M. G. and KOPIN, I. J. *Life Sci.,* **18,** 1315 (1976)
24. VARGAS, E. and LYE, M. *Age Ageing,* **9**, 210 (1980)
25. GRIBBIN, B., PICKERING, T. G., SLEIGHT, P. and PETO, R. *Circulation Res.,* **29**, 424 (1971)
26. VARGAS, E. and LYE, M. *Exper. Gerontol.,* **17**, 445 (1982)
27. VARGAS, E., LYE, M., FARAGHER, E. B. *et al. Age Ageing,* **15**, 17 (1986)
28. ROBINSON, B. J., JOHNSON, R. H., LAMBIE, D. G. and PALMER, K. T. *Clin. Sci.,* **64**, 587 (1983)
29. LIPSITZ, L. A., PLUCHINO, F. C., WEI, J. Y. *et al. Am. J. Cardiol.,* **58**, 810 (1986)
30. BRADSHAW, M. J. and EDWARDS, R. T. M. *Q. J. Med.,* **60**, 643 (1986)
31. CAMPBELL, A. J. and REINKEN, J. *J. Clin. Exper. Gerontol.,* **7**, 163 (1985)
32. LYE, M. *Clin. Endocrinol. Metabol.,* **13**, 377 (1984)
33. SHY, G. M. AND DRAGER, G. A. *Arch. Neurol.,* **2**, 511 (1960)
34. PATRI, B. *Therapie,* **40**, 41 (1985)
36. WARREN, L. R., BUTLER, R. W., KATHOLI, C. R. and HALSEY, J. H. *J. Gerontol.,* **40**, 53 (1985)
37. CLARK, C. V. and MAPSTONE, R. *Age Ageing,* **15**, 221 (1986)
38. HAINSWORTH, R. and AL-SHAMMA, Y. M. H. *Clin. Sci.,* **74**, 17 (1988)
39. KAIJISER, L. and SACHS, C. *Clin. Physiol.,* **5**, 347 (1985)
40. PARNATI, G., POMIDOSSI, G., RAMIREZ, A. *et al. Clin. Sci.,* **69**, 533 (1985)
41. WATSON, R. D. S. *Br. Med. J.,* **294**, 390 (1987)
42. GOOVAERTS, J., VERFAILLIE, C., FAGARD, R. and KNOCKAERT, D. *Br. Med. J.,* **288**, 817 (1984)
43. BOBIK, A., JENNINGS, G., SKEWS, H. *et al. Clin. Pharmacol. Ther.,* **30**, 673 (1981)
44. IMAIZUMI, T., TAKESHITA, A., ASHIHARA, T. *et al. Br. Heart J.,* **52**, 581 (1984)
45. LEVY, D. W. and LYE, M. *J. R. Coll. Phys. (Lond.),* **21**, 148 (1987)
46. BENA, A. M. *Clin. Pharmacol. Ther.,* **36**, 738 (1984)
47. ORME, M. L. E. and TALLIS, R. C. *Br. Med. J.,* **289**, 397 (1984)
48. YAMASHITA, M. *Lancet,* **1**, 1431 (1987)
49. WILLIAMS, T. D . M., DA COSTA, D., MATHIAS, C. J. *et al. Clin. Sci.,* **71**, 173 (1986)
50. KIRKLAND, J. L., LYE, M., GODDARD, C. *et al. Clin. Endocrinol.,* **20**, 451 (1984)

Chapter 7

Epilepsy in the elderly

R. C. Tallis

An epileptic fit is always a terrifying experience, and to an elderly patient such an attack may seem a harbinger of death. For this reason explanation and reassurance are all-important aspects of medical care. The general principles of management are essentially the same as in younger patients. The first step is to determine whether or not the event is epileptic. The next is to consider the possibility that the seizures are symptomatic of an underlying cause. This is particularly likely when fits occur for the first time in an elderly person. If an underlying cause is identified, this may require treatment in its own right. The next step will be control of the fits, if recurrent, usually by drug treatment. Finally it will be necessary to monitor control of fits, to watch for the emergence of new pointers as to any underlying cause that may need treatment and to ensure that the patient is not disabled by adverse drug reactions.

So much is clear. Nevertheless there are many unanswered questions about epilepsy in old age; estimates of frequency vary; views as to the relative frequency of different causes are changing; the appropriate first-line anticonvulsant is yet to be established; and we are still in the process of learning elementary facts about the pharmacokinetics and pharmacodynamics of anticonvulsants in this age group.

Epidemiology

The incidence of new cases rises steeply with age above 50. Hauser and Kurland[1] found that the annual incidence of epileptic seizures rose from 11.9 per 100 000 in the 40–59 age range to 82 per 100 000 in those over 60. A more recent Danish study[2], which included all patients over 60 in a well-defined population who developed epilepsy during a 5-year period, found an incidence of 77 per 100 000 new cases per year. Estimates of prevalence are more difficult because of the tendency of epilepsy to remit, though this occurs less often in older subjects in whom fits tend to be symptomatic. Hauser and Kurland[1] found an increase in the prevalence from 7.3 per 1000 in the 40–59 age range to 10.2 for those over 60.

Diagnosis

This may be more difficult in the elderly in whom syncopal attacks are more common and hypoglycaemic drugs often prescribed. Moreover, many elderly people live alone and an adequate history with good eye-witness reports may not be available. The findings on examination and investigations, even sophisticated ones such as ambulatory ECG and EEG, may raise more questions than they answer[3]. Even after intensive investigation and monitoring it is often not possible to be sure whether 'funny dos' originate from the heart or the head. Where fits are frequent, admission for observation may be the most helpful investigation.

Types of fit

Hildick-Smith[4] pointed out that series originating from neuromedical centres may have a bias. One obvious bias is likely to be the under-representation of the elderly and certainly of the unfit elderly typically encountered by geriatricians. In Hildick-Smith's series of 50 patients (mean age 79), 28 had grand mal attacks, 12 had focal attacks and 7 had both. EEG findings were not reported. Roberts *et al.*[5] studied 81 patients over 65, again without EEG correlation. Sixty-five percent had grand mal seizures and 25% partial seizures only. Although these two geriatric series give a lower percentage of focal seizures than many other adult series, this difference may be due to a lack of EEG information. This interpretation is supported by the survey of Luhdorf *et al.*[2], who reported on 163 new elderly patients in their 5-year study. Of these, 51% had grand mal seizures, 42% had partial or secondary generalized seizures and 10% were unclassified. Of those with grand mal seizures, however, 38% had focal abnormalities on the EEG.

Neuropsychiatric presentations of epilepsy in the elderly may present diagnostic problems. Simple partial seizures associated with disturbances of higher cerebral function, or complex partial seizures with or without automatism, may be labelled as non-specific confusional states or, where there are affective or cognitive features or hallucinations, as manifestations of functional psychiatric illnesses. This is particularly likely to occur in patients with non-convulsive epileptic status[6]. Ellis and Lee[7] described 6 late-middle-aged patients who presented with acute behavioural changes – withdrawal, mutism, delusional ideas, paranoia and vivid hallucinations. All 6 had generalized spike and wave discharges and all responded well to anticonvulsants. Andermann and Robb[8] recommend the term 'absence status' for such patients rather than 'petit mal', which is more specifically associated with 3/s spike and wave discharges and is a condition of childhood.

Godfrey *et al.*[9] draw attention to the fact that post-ictal confusion may be very prolonged in the elderly, in some cases persisting for up to a week. Post-ictal paresis (Todd's palsy) is also common in the elderly and is especially likely to occur in patients with post-stroke epilepsy as Fine[10,11] has pointed out, when it may be mistaken for a further stroke. Moreover, post-ictal hemiparesis was the commonest cause for erroneous referral to a stroke unit in a review by Norris and Hachinski on the misdiagnosis of stroke[12].

Somatosensory epilepsy is rare[13] but may cause diagnostic difficulties. Most patients have paraesthesiae of short duration, usually of the hand and upper limb. This may be confused with transient ischaemic attacks or, in those patients who have episodic pain following stroke, other causes of post-stroke pain.

Very localized motor status (epilepsia partialis continua) is sometimes misdiagnosed as an extrapyramidal movement disorder[14]. It tends to be of a sudden onset and can be highly variable in the same patient.

Epileptic dizziness, consisting of a sensation of disequilibrium, often with a sense of rotation, has recently been reviewed in younger patients by Kogeorgos *et al.*[15]. The episodes typically consisted of brief periods of dizziness, often lasting no more than a few seconds, followed sometimes by nausea. Attacks may be very frequent and a quarter of the patients had generalized convulsions by the time of referral. Half of them had suffered brief absences. Less commonly, there were other temporal lobe features. Anticonvulsant treatment is very effective.

Aetiology of late onset epilepsy

As can be seen from Table 7.1, cerebrovascular disease is by far the commonest cause of late onset epilepsy, accounting for up to 60% of cases in which a cause is found. The relationship between

Table 7.1 Causes of epilepsy in the elderly as reported in the literature

	Series			
	Hildick-Smith [4] %	*Schold [20]* %	*Godfrey [9]* %	*Luhdorf [2]* %
Cerebrovascular disease	42(48)	30(60)	44(52)	32
Cerebral tumour	10	2	12	14
Senile dementia/ cerebral atrophy	14		7	2
Toxic/metabolic	12	10	6	12

Figures in brackets are percentages of those cases in which a cause was found

epilepsy and cerebrovascular disease has also been studied the other way round. Marquardsen[16] noted epilepsy occurring in 8% of hemiplegic stroke patients. Cocito *et al.*[17] examined the incidence of post-stroke epilepsy in patients with angiographically proved carotid or middle cerebral artery occlusive disease and found that fits occurred in 17.3% of carotid patients and 10.8% of middle cerebral artery patients. Most seizures were partial motor attacks. Shorvon *et al.*[18] compared the CT-scan appearances of 74 patients with late onset epilepsy and no evidence of cerebral tumours with those of age- and sex-matched controls. There was an excess of ischaemic lesions in epileptic patients. In half of the epileptic patients who were found to have CT evidence of vascular disease, clinical examination was normal. Finally, Shinton *et al.*[19] found an excess of previous epilepsy in patients admitted to hospital with acute stroke compared with controls.

Other cerebral causes of epilepsy are less common. Hildick-Smith[4] and Roberts *et al.*[5] found cerebral tumours in 10% and 12% respectively of their cases. The much lower figure of 2% in the series of Schold *et al.*[20] is less reliable because in nearly 50% of cases no cause was found. Luhdorf *et al.*[2] found tumours in 14%. Of these all but one were either metastases or inoperable gliomas. The percentage of seizures associated with non-vascular cerebral degeneration is uncertain and will remain so until large series with uniform access to CT scanning facilities are reported. Subdural haematoma is a rare but important remediable cause. Finally, seizures may rarely occur in severe cerebral infections or following recovery from such infections due to scarring.

As can be seen from Table 7.1, toxic and metabolic causes are important factors in epilepsy of old age. In Luhdorf's series, 12% of cases were attributed to drugs, alcohol or metabolic disturbances[2]. Dam[21] found that alcohol or alcohol withdrawal was the main cause in 25% of patients with late onset epilepsy. Moreover, alcohol appeared to be the sole precipitating factor in 20% of cases of status epilepticus in the series of Pilke *et al.*[22].

Many other metabolic disturbances may precipitate fits in the elderly person; these include uraemia, hepatic failure, myxoedema, hypoxia, hypercapnoea, hypoglycaemia, hypocalcaemia, hyponatraemia and water intoxication. Uraemia seems to be the commonest of these in most series.

Drug-induced epilepsy

More than 70 drugs have been suspected of causing convulsions. These include anaesthetic agents, analgesics, steroids, antibiotics, hypnotics, tranquillizers and antidepressants[23]. Drug-induced seizures are most likely to occur when the drug is given in high dosage, parenterally or to patients with impaired drug metabolism or excretion. Aminophylline, which has a narrow therapeutic index, and whose disposition may be inhibited by cigarette smoking, is particularly prone to cause generalized seizures[24].

Idiopathic

Some patients presenting with epilepsy apparently for the first time in old age will in fact be suffering from a recurrence of earlier idiopathic epilepsy or, indeed, may have a long history of epilepsy which has not been recognized.

Investigations

The traditional emphasis on remediable structural underlying causes is based on an exaggerated estimate of the frequency with which tumours are the cause of late onset epilepsy, the percentage of such tumours that are benign or amenable to neurosurgical removal and an underestimate of the importance of other neurological or, more significantly, metabolic causes. Nevertheless, modern methods of neurological investigation are relatively benign and it is easy to undervalue the benefit of having a precise diagnosis of the underlying cause even where this may not be amenable to definitive treatment.

General investigations

The investigations will be guided by the history and findings on examination and by a consideration of the likely causes, which will include metabolic disturbances. An estimate of gamma glutamyl transferase may be a useful marker of alcohol consumption. Diabetic patients on treatment should have their control reviewed. If it is suspected that fits are secondary to syncope, carotid sinus massage and ambulatory ECG may be considered. In the absence of definite pointers to infectious disease of the nervous system there is no indication for lumbar puncture.

Electroencephalography

The most commonly misunderstood investigation is the electroencephalogram (EEG). A routine EEG may support the diagnosis of epilepsy, especially if clear-cut paroxysmal discharges are observed. Nevertheless, the absence of inter-ictal or epileptogenic activity on a 20 min recording does not rule out this diagnosis. Moreover, the EEG changes with age, so that discriminating significant from insignificant findings becomes more difficult. A focal abnormality on the EEG may support the diagnosis of a focal origin for fits and suggest a local neurological cause. In those fits where there is an inadequate history or where the focal phase is too brief to be observed clinically before generalization, the suggestion of a focal origin may be raised for the first time by an EEG. Thus, the EEG may provide invaluable supporting evidence for the diagnosis and suggest the need for further examination, but it should rarely overrule the clinical diagnosis. It cannot determine the need for treatment in a newly diagnosed case, establish the adequacy of treatment or predict the safety of withdrawing anticonvulsants.

Neuroradiology

Isotope brain scanning may now be considered obsolete except in those centres without access to computerized tomography (CT). If all elderly patients who had fits were automatically referred for CT scanning, the burden on the service would be overwhelming. The presence of focal neurological signs, a history of head injury and the absence of evidence of a metabolic or toxic cause will strengthen the case for a scan, particularly if the patient's general health is good. The case will be particularly strong in patients who have progressive neurological signs or features suggestive of raised intracranial pressure.

The diagnostic yield of CT scanning in epilepsy has been the subject of many recent studies[25–27]. All these show that scanning increases the frequency with which a definitive diagnosis is obtained. The study of Ramirez-Lassepas's team is particularly relevant to the elderly. Excluding patients with known tumours, craniotomy, open skull fracture and a history of alcoholism, they found a cause for seizures in 48% of cases and established a structural lesion by CT scanning in 37% of the total series. There was a marked rise in abnormal scans with age and there was a much higher percentage of positive scans in patients with focal seizures. Interestingly, just over one-third of the positive scans were seen in patients with no focal features or focal findings, and generalized rather than focal abnormalities on the EEG.

Some authors have questioned the value of the increased information obtained by CT scanning. Young *et al.*[26] pointed out that only one-quarter of the abnormalities detected by CT scanning were potentially treatable by surgery and less than 10% of patients had their management changed as a result of CT scanning. In addition, 3 out of the 11 patients with tumours initially had a normal scan. They conclude that routine scanning is inappropriate, that it should be reserved for patients with focal features and that a negative scan should not be sought for reassurance. Other clinicians may interpret these findings differently; as so often in medicine, decisions reflect personal judgement. The threshold for scanning will depend at least in part on the available resources, but scanning should not necessarily be ruled out simply on the ground that the chances of finding an operable lesion are slim.

Treatment

The general management of an elderly patient with epilepsy is similar to that of younger patients. The explanation of the condition is of paramount importance and this, along with a reassurance that in the great majority of cases the seizures are unpleasant rather than dangerous and that they can be controlled, is crucial. Patients should be advised against activities that would mean immediate danger if a fit occurred. Factors that are known to precipitate fits, such as sleep deprivation, excess alcohol intake and sudden alcohol withdrawal in heavy drinkers, should be avoided. Patients should be warned that the side-effects of anticonvulsants will be increased by alcohol and they will also need to be advised of the regulations regarding driving. These have recently been reviewed[28].

Initiating treatment

Most patients who have had a single grand mal seizure are 'let off with a caution' rather than being put on anticonvulsant treatment straightaway. Studies of the prognosis of a single grand mal fit, however, have shown a recurrence rate of over 60% by one year[29]. One would expect this figure to be higher in elderly patients, in whom there is a high proportion of cases associated with cerebral disease. Since the risks attending an epileptic fit are increased in this age group, there would appear to be a case for treating a first tonic-clonic seizure. There is no information about the prognosis for untreated minor seizures but as the problems associated with treatment are liable to be greater in the elderly it may be reasonable to 'wait and see' unless there is clear clinical or CT scanning evidence of a focal lesion.

Monotherapy or polytherapy?

The fashion for putting epileptic patients on a multitude of anticonvulsants in subtherapeutic or toxic doses has now passed as a result of the careful studies and persuasive advocacy of Reynolds and his co-workers. The disadvantages of polytherapy are self evident and have been summarized by Reynolds *et al.*[30]. Moreover, it has been shown that most patients can be adequately controlled on a single drug[30–32]. Where monotherapy has failed there is little evidence that the introduction of a second drug contributes anything to the management of the patient other than increasing the risk of side-effects[33].

The choice of drug

The main drugs to be considered in the elderly are phenytoin, carbamazepine and sodium valproate – which are all broad spectrum anticonvulsants. The studies already mentioned have demonstrated the effectiveness of phenytoin monotherapy in both generalized and partial seizures. Unfortunately this is a drug with many side-effects and, although these may be reduced by careful serum monitoring, they may still be troublesome in the elderly. Carbamazepine is also effective in most forms of epilepsy that are seen in the elderly. A small double-blind cross-over study[34] comparing phenytoin and carbamazepine in patients with both grand mal and focal motor seizures showed no difference in the efficacy or side-effects of these two drugs. Phenytoin, however, has a better defined therapeutic range.

One of the most interesting developments in recent years has been the increasing use of sodium valproate – originally introduced for primary generalized epilepsy – in partial and secondary generalized fits. Turnbull *et al.*[35] randomized 140 previously untreated patients with tonic-clonic or partial seizures to receive either phenytoin or sodium valproate. There was no difference in the efficacy of the two drugs, irrespective of the type of seizures suffered, during a follow-up period of 2–4 years. Adverse reactions were more common in patients on phenytoin. It is possible then that sodium valproate may become the drug of first choice for most seizures in the elderly. Chadwick and Turnbull[36] point out that there are large deficits in the literature and that the strong feelings clinicians have about the choice of first-line drugs are not based on adequate information.

It used to be traditional to give anticonvulsants three times a day. This is irrational in the case of phenytoin, which has a long half-life of 24–48 hours[37]. There is now evidence that a single daily dose of phenytoin is as effective as divided doses and has no increased adverse effects[38]. As yet no comparable studies have been carried out with carbamazepine or sodium valproate and the recommended frequency is two or three divided doses daily. The rate of phenytoin metabolism is decreased in elderly patients and it has been estimated that they require 20% less phenytoin than in younger patients to maintain the same steady state concentration[39]. It has been suggested that a lower starting dose (200 mg total daily dose) should be employed. The best guide to optimal dosage is the clinical response and anticonvulsant levels. Without monitoring levels, failure to respond to treatment may lead to inappropriate or premature change of medication. Moreover, in the case of phenytoin, the therapeutic ratio is very narrow and there is therefore an increased chance of straying outside the therapeutic range. There is a clear relationship between phenytoin levels and both therapeutic effects and toxicity. This relationship is less well defined for sodium valproate. It is not possible to determine the therapeutic range of carbamazepine as a wide range of levels is associated with efficacy and side-effects[31].

The saturation kinetics of phenytoin mean that the relationship between the dose and the steady state is not linear. For this reason, smaller increments, e.g. 25 mg are recommended[40]. Increments of 50 or 100 mg may result in a swing from a subtherapeutic to a toxic dose. The optimum plasma levels of anticonvulsants have not yet been studied separately for the elderly. In view of the higher incidence of cerebral impairment due to age-related changes and cerebral diseases in the elderly epileptic population, one might expect increased pharmaco-dynamic sensitivity.

Side-effects

The most important side-effects of anticonvulsants are neuro-psychiatric and these have recently been comprehensively reviewed by Trimble and Reynolds[41]. Sodium valproate appears to cause fewer neuropsychiatric disturbances than phenytoin; carbamazepine may have an intermediate position. Other side-effects relate to the gastrointestinal system, the bones and blood and skin. Sodium valproate appears to produce hepatic dysfunction and for this reason its use is usually avoided in patients with existing liver impairment. Hepatic failure has been described mainly in very young children, who may have metabolic defects, but further research is needed before the recommendation to avoid sodium valproate in the presence of hepatic dysfunction can be revised.

The numerous interactions in anticonvulsants and other drugs are usefully listed in Appendix 1 of the British National Formulary.

Can anticonvulsants be stopped?

Studies of withdrawal of anticonvulsants have shown that up to 40% of patients free of seizures for 2 years or more may relapse in the 2–5 years after withdrawal from treatment[42,43]. The chances of withdrawal are increased by an increasing age of the patient and in partial seizures. This latter is probably correlated with the fact that the presence of known cerebral pathology increases the rate of relapse. In view of the fact that in many elderly patients seizures are related to cerebral pathology, the chances of successfully withdrawing medication are remote.

References

1. HAUSER, A. and KURLAND, L. T. *Epilepsia*, **16**, 1–66 (1975)
2. LUHDORF, K., JENSEN, L. K. and PLESNER, A. *Epilepsia*, **27**, 458–463 (1986)
3. BLUMHARDT, L. D. *Br. J. Hosp. Med.*, **36**, 354–360 (1986)
4. HILDICK-SMITH, M. *Age Ageing*, **3**, 203–208 (1974)
5. ROBERTS, M. A., GODFREY, J. W. and CAIRD, F. I. *Age Ageing*, **11**, 24–28 (1982)
6. DRAKE, M. E. and COFFEY, C. E. *Am. J. Psychiat.*, **140**, 800–801 (1983)
7. ELLIS, J. M. and LEE, S. I. *Epilepsia*, **19**, 119–128 (1978)
8. ANDERMANN, F. and ROBB, J. P. *Epilepsia*, **13**, 17 (1972)
9. GODFREY, J. W., ROBERTS, M. A. and CAIRD, F. I. *Age Ageing*, **11**, 29–34 (1982)
10. FINE, W. *Clin. Gerontol.*, **8**, 21–33 (1966)
11. FINE, W. *Br. Med. J.*, **1**, 199–201 (1967)

12. NORRIS, J. W. and HACHINSKI, V. C. *Lancet,* **1**, 328–331 (1982)
13. MAGUIERE, F. and COUJON, J. *Brain,* **101**, 307–332 (1978)
14. THOMAS, J. E., REAGAN, T. J. and KLASS, D. W. *Arch. Neurol.,* **34**, 266–275 (1977)
15. KOGEORGOS, J., SCOTT, D. F. and SWASH, M. *Br. Med. J. (Clin. Res.),* **282**, 687–689 (1981)
16. MARQUARDSEN, J. *Acta Neurol. Scand.,* **45** (Suppl. 38), 150–152 (1969)
17. COCITO, L., FAVALE, E. and RENI, L. *Stroke,* **13**, 189–195 (1982)
18. SHORVON, S. D., GILLIATT, R. W., COX, T. C. and YU, Y. L. *J. Neurol. Neurosurg. Psychiat.,* **47**, 225–230 (1984)
19. SHINTON, R. A., GILL, J. S., ZEZULK, A. V. and BEEVERS, D. J. *Lancet,* **1**, 11–13 (1987)
20. SCHOLD, C., WARNELL, P. R. and EARNEST, N. P. *JAMA,* **238**, 1177–1178 (1977)
21. DAM, A. M. *Epilepsia,* **26**, 227–231 (1985)
22. PILKE, A., PARTINEN, M. and KOVANEN, J. *Acta Neurol. Scand.,* **70**, 443–450 (1984)
23. CHADWICK, D. W. *Adv. Drug React. Bull.,* **87**, 316–319 (1981)
24. YARNELL, P. R. and CHU, N. S. *Neurology (Minneap),* **25**, 819–822 (1975)
25. GASTAUT, H. and GASTAUT, J. L. *Epilepsia,* **17**, 326–336 (1976)
26. YOUNG, A. C., COSTANZI, J. B., MOHR, P. D. and FORBES, W. S. *Lancet,* **2**, 1446–1447 (1982)
27. RAMIREZ-LASSEPAS, M., CIPOLLE, R. J., MORILLO, L. R. and GUMNIT, R. J. *Ann. Neurol.,* **15**, 436–443 (1984)
28. ESPIR, M. L. E. *Health Trends,* **15**, 46–47 (1983)
29. ELWES, R. D., JOHNSON, A. L., SHORVON, S. D. and REYNOLDS, E. H. *N. Engl. J. Med.,* **311**, 944–947 (1984)
30. REYNOLDS, E. H., SHORVON, S. D., GALBRAITH, A. W. *et al. Epilepsia,* **22**, 475–488 (1981)
31. CALLAGHAN, N., O'CALLAGHAN, M., DUGGAN, B. and FEELY, M. *J. Neurol. Neurosurg. Psychiat.,* **41**, 907–912 (1978)
32. ANDERSEN, E. B., PHILBERT, A. and KLEE, J. G. *Acta Neurol. Scand.,* **94** (Suppl.), 29–34 (1983)
33. SHORVON, S. D. and REYNOLDS, E. H. *Br. Med. J.,* **1**, 1635–1637 (1977)
34. KOSTELJANETZ, M., CHRISTIANSEN, J., DAM, A. M. *et al. Arch. Neurol.,* **36**, 22–24 (1979)
35. TURNBULL, D. M., HOWELL, D., RAWLINS, M. D. *et al. Br. Med. J.,* **290**, 815–819 (1985)
36. CHADWICK, D. and TURNBULL, D. M. *J. Neurol. Neurosurg. Psychiat.,* **48**, 1073–1077 (1985)
37. WOODBURY, D. M. In *Anti-epileptic Drugs* (ed. D. M. Woodbury, J. K. Penry and C. E. Pippinger), Raven Press, New York, p. 191 (1982)
38. O'DRISCOLL, K., GHADIALI, E., CRAWFORD, P. and CHADWICK, D. *Acta Ther.,* **11**, 375–385 (1985)
39. BAUER, L. A. and BLOUIN, R. A. *Clin. Pharmacol. Ther.,* **31**, 301–304 (1982)
40. MAWER, G. E., MULLEN, P. W., RODGERS, M. *et al. Br. J. Clin. Pharmacol.,* **1**, 163–168 (1974)
41. TRIMBLE, M. R. and REYNOLDS, E. H. In *Recent Advances in Clinical Neurology,* vol. 4 (ed. W. B. Matthews and G. H. Glaser), Churchill Livingstone, Edinburgh, p. 261 (1983)
42. CHADWICK, D. In *Dilemmas in the Management of the Neurological Patient* (ed. C. Warlow and J. Garfield), Churchill Livingstone, Edinburgh, p. 133 (1984)
43. JUUL-JENSEN, P. *Epilepsia,* **9**, 11–16 (1968)

Chapter 8

The transient global amnesia syndrome

J. R. Hodges

Transient global amnesia (TGA) is now a well-established clinical syndrome. More than 1000 cases have been reported, and yet it remains an enigma. The underlying pathogenesis is unknown, the aetiology controversial and the natural history uncertain. Over the past few years the present author has been involved in a large epidemiological and neuropsychological study of TGA patients. This chapter is based on a review of the literature and a personal study of more than 100 cases.

First descriptions of transient global amnesia

In 1958 Fisher and Adams[1] reported 12 patients with a distinct and stereotyped clinical syndrome, which they felt had not been clearly described in the medical literature. They termed this syndrome 'transient global amnesia'. Six years later the same authors published a much more extensive account of 17 cases of TGA[2]. Their patients, who were middle aged or elderly and in good health, suddenly experienced an episode of profound memory loss lasting a few hours. Many of the attacks were witnessed by relatives or family doctors, and two patients were examined by neurologists during the episode. During the attack the patients were unable to retain new information for more than a few moments. This profound learning deficit, often manifested by repetitive questioning, was accompanied by a variable length of retrograde amnesia for events days, weeks, months or even years prior to the attack. Personal identity was preserved and consciousness clear throughout. There were no associated automatisms or epileptic aura. No disturbance of motor power, coordination or speech was noted. After approximately 2–8 hours the period of retrograde amnesia gradually shrank and the patients became lucid. There persisted a dense amnesic gap for the period between the onset and termination of the attack. The authors noted a number of unusual precipitating influences, including 'bathing in the cool waters of the Atlantic off the New England coast', sexual intercourse and 'shower baths'.

The recurrence rate over many years of follow-up was low and the general prognosis good. All routine investigations, including EEGs, were normal. Because of the lack of vascular risk factors, the lack of accompanying clinical features to indicate ischaemia in the posterior circulation and the low recurrence rate, Fisher and Adams concluded that ischaemia of the ordinary cerebrovascular variety played no part in the aetiology and that, although the attacks were unassociated with overt epilepsy, most evidence was consistent with cerebral seizure activity. In view of subsequent authors' use of the term TGA, it should be stressed that in their original description of the syndrome, Fisher and Adams explicitly separated TGA from epilepsy and excluded patients with focal neurological deficits or other cognitive problems during the attack.

The syndrome was almost certainly described by other authors but under different titles. Bender[3,4] coined the term 'isolated episode of confusion with amnesia'. He stressed 'the singleness of the attack without recurrence over a period of years'. He considered vascular disease, post-convulsive confusion, toxic-metabolic states and hysteria as possible aetiologies and concluded that although all explanations were inadequate, perhaps a transient circulatory disturbance of the brain would be the most acceptable. In the French literature an identical syndrome was reported under the title of 'L'ictus amnésique'. Guyotat and Courjon[5] were the first to apply this term, which later became popular[6,7]. They too favoured a cerebrovascular aetiology in their report of 16 cases with 'a disturbance of consciousness affecting principally amnesic functions occurring suddenly and lasting for only a short period of time'. Haas[8] should be credited for bringing attention to what is probably the earliest definite description of TGA, by Hauge in 1954. The latter author included in a monograph on the complications of vertebral angiography, three cases with amnesia, as 'the only demonstrable symptom' after the procedure.

TGA in the early twentieth century

Considering the number of reported cases of TGA since the original descriptions in the 1950s and 1960s, it is remarkable that this distinct and characteristic syndrome escaped the notice of clinicians for so long. It seems inconceivable that it arose as a new entity in the 1950s, so why did the great neurologists of the late nineteenth and early twentieth century not recognize TGA? It seems most likely that the syndrome is immersed in the psychiatric literature on amnesia. Prior to the description of TGA, most cases of isolated sudden memory loss were considered to be due to hysteria or malingering. After the First World War the diagnosis of hysterical amnesia became extremely common. An extraordinary number of cases were reported right up until the 1960s; for instance, Kanzer[9] reported 71 cases of amnesia seen in a single year at the Bellevue Hospital, New York, including several who were aged over 60 years. Since the early 1960s there have been very few reports of hysterical amnesia and it seems a strange coincidence that hysterical amnesia should suddenly become so uncommon since the description of TGA.

Establishment of the syndrome

Within a few years of Fisher and Adams's monograph[2], the term TGA had gained ascendancy over other proposed titles for the syndrome. A steady stream of case reports followed and by the end of the 1970s approximately 200 cases had been reported, including descriptions from most Western countries. This trickle of reports was followed by a flood, so that by 1987 there were more than 1000 reported cases in the literature. Clearly TGA is not a rare syndrome. The author's clinic in Oxford has now studied 114 cases referred over an 8 year period. The estimated incidence is in the order of 5 per 100 000 per year, although the majority of cases are probably never seen in hospital.

Despite the mass of literature, little has been learned about the basic underlying mechanism of the syndrome. The elegant clinical descriptions by the early authors have not been bettered. There have been some advances in understanding the neuropsychology of TGA and a small number of cases have now been studied more formally during an attack[10–12]. However, while the characteristics are quite clear (see Table 8.1), it is the aetiology that has continued to be the major focus of interest and debate.

Table 8.1 Characteristic features of TGA

Patients usually elderly (55–85 years)
Abrupt onset of profound anterograde amnesia
Variable retrograde amnesia
Often repetitive questioning
Retention of personal identity
No clouding of consciousness
Absence of *focal* neurological deficits
Resolution within 24 hours
Complete amnesic gap for duration of attack

Putative pathology: the anatomy of memory

Whatever the pathogenesis of TGA, all agree that the area of brain involved must be the deep mid-line structures of the limbic system and that the severity of memory disturbance argues for bilateral pathology. Clinicopathological studies in permanent amnesic subjects have identified where damage must occur to produce severe memory loss: the medial temporal region (with emphasis on hippocampus) and the diencephalic structures, which surround the third ventricle (of these the mammillary bodies and the dorsomedial nuclei of the thalamus appear most important). Between these two major areas there are rich connections via the fornix, cingulate and basal forebrain. Together, these structures constitute what is sometimes called the circle of Papez. The exact role of each of the structures is a topic of fierce debate between experimental neuropsychologists[13,14]. Surgical extirpation of unilateral temporal lobe structures results in a minor degree of memory disturbance – a verbal memory deficit in the case of left temporal lobectomy and non-verbal memory in the case of right temporal lobe surgery. Only after bilateral damage or surgery does a profound amnesic syndrome result[16].

The blood supply of these structures is complex. The anterior hippocampus, amygdala and mammillary bodies derive some blood from the internal carotid artery via the anterior choroidal artery, but the majority of the structures, including the vital dorsomedial nucleus of the thalamus, most of the hippocampus and parahippocampal gyrus are supplied by branches of the posterior cerebral artery[15].

The importance of considering the blood supply to these areas is obvious. If thromboembolic cerebrovascular disease were to be responsible for TGA, then the expected site of vascular pathology would be in the vertebrobasilar system. The blood supply of the memory structures is also relevant to the proposed role of migraine in the pathogenesis of TGA. There is clinical and laboratory evidence that posterior circulatory disturbances occur during migraine attacks, which have been linked with amnesia[17].

Precipitating factors

Any consideration of the aetiology of TGA should take into account the extraordinary number of reports of cases apparently associated with unusual provoking or precipitating factors. These include:

1. Immersion in cold water, especially the sea – a phenomenon referred to as 'amnesia at the seaside'[18]. Similarly, attacks following hot or cold baths and showers have been mentioned on several occasions[19].
2. Sexual intercourse – a number of patients with attacks during or shortly following coitus have been described[19–22].
3. Physical exertion – exertion ranging from digging, chopping wood, gymnastics or yoga, raking snow and pedalling a bicycle has apparently precipitated attacks[19–23].
4. Painful experiences – such as dental extraction, abdominal pain or trigeminal nerve stimulation[19,24].
5. Emotional stress – a number of authors have drawn attention to the occurrence of TGA following periods of particular emotional stress. Examples are, attending a very ill husband, a visit to a cemetery, an important job interview, the recent death of a sister, witnessing a husband's sudden death, receiving an obscene telephone call, discussing a son's recent suicide and signing a document authorizing state confiscation of a family business[17,19,25,26].

The role of such factors remains unclear. In our study of 114 cases, 3% occurred after swimming, 3% followed sexual intercourse and 5%, medical procedures. In addition, 11% reported an emotionally stressful event during the preceding 24 hours.

6. Angiography – a total of 30 cases have now been reported following cerebral angiography, usually of the vertebral artery[27–29]. Emboli from atheromatous debris or catheter clot, secondary to catheter manipulation problems, was suggested as a possible cause. In addition to the cases complicating cerebral angiography, examples of TGA occurring during or shortly after cardiac angiograms have been reported[30]. It should be noted that overall, angiography is a very rare cause of TGA. We have seen no such examples among our 114 cases.

Diagnostic criteria

In studying any disease it is vital that the diagnostic criteria are strictly defined. This is particularly so when considering a condition like TGA, which is defined entirely on clinical grounds, and for which the diagnosis cannot be verified by laboratory investigations. Examination of the literature reveals that there is no consistent use of the diagnosis and that the vast majority of authors have given no criteria.

Fisher and Adams[2] did not stipulate criteria, but they were specific and selective in the use of the term, to include only patients with well-documented acute amnesia, without other cognitive deficits, focal, neurological or epileptic phenomena. Patients with epilepsy or recent head injury were excluded, as were those with residual neurological signs or permanent memory loss after the attack. Many subsequent authors have applied the diagnosis very loosely, to include a variety of clinical situations merely showing the feature of prominent memory loss. As a result the original carefully considered diagnosis has been widened and corrupted. It is, therefore, not surprising that so much controversy exists regarding the aetiology and natural history of the condition.

As there are no generally accepted diagnostic criteria, I reviewed the literature, looking specifically at the use of the diagnostic terms and criteria where given. Based on this review and the diagnostic guidelines laid down by Caplan[31], I have delineated what I consider to be the essential clinical components of the syndrome and accordingly propose strict diagnostic criteria.

1. Eye-witness reporting of attack   It is well known that a period of amnesia and confusion may follow seizures, especially of temporal lobe type, and that head injury causes persistent retrograde and anterograde amnesia, so that patients' recall of the cause of injury may be erased. If attacks of amnesia go unwitnessed these cases cannot be reasonably excluded. In addition, only observation of patients during an attack can diagnose hysterical or feigned amnesia. The first essential must therefore be that the attack is witnessed by a capable observer, from whom an accurate report can be obtained.

2. Clear-cut evidence of anterograde amnesia during the attack
Patients who remain normal but who later report a memory gap do not qualify.

3. Absence of other cognitive deficits and focal neurological features   Amnesia is an integral part of acute confusional states which must be separated from TGA. Evidence of general cognitive impairment or clouding of consciousness is clearly grounds for exclusion. The inclusion of patients with focal neurological features within the rubric of TGA is likely to have a major impact on considerations of aetiology and natural history of the syndrome. On the whole, those authors whose studies include cases with additional neurological features have supported a cerebrovascular aetiology, whereas those using stricter criteria have rejected this hypothesis. I propose that the diagnosis should be reserved for cases without focal neurological symptoms or signs.

4. Duration: resolution within 24 hours   Inherent in the title of the syndrome is the transient nature of the memory loss. Clearly, patients with persisting amnesia do not qualify for the diagnosis. Any time limit is purely arbitrary, but it would seem reasonable to adopt the same terminology as that used in cerebrovascular disease and to limit the use of the term TGA to attacks lasting less than 24 hours. In our series the median duration was 3.5 hours and the longest 12 hours. Attacks of less than 1 hour's duration are unusual and should be regarded with caution, as patients with such brief attacks have a high rate of subsequent epilepsy.

5. Exclusion categories   Recently, Haas and Ross[32] used the term TGA in association with a group of nine young patients (11–28 years), who became acutely amnesic after mild head injury. Other authors have included cases with known epilepsy. I propose that subjects with known active epilepsy or recent head injuries be excluded.

I have studied 114 definite TGA cases fulfilling strict criteria and 39 others whose attacks were poorly witnessed or had additional features. There was good evidence that the criteria selected a homogenous population with a very good prognosis. Cases who did not fulfil the criteria had a worse prognosis and 15% developed overt epilepsy on follow-up.

Aetiology

Cerebrovascular disease

The most prevalent and widely accepted view is that TGA is due to cerebrovascular disease of thromboembolic type. This aetiology is favoured by the vast majority of authors and is stated in the standard medical and neurological textbooks. Adams and Victor conclude in their *Principles of Neurology*[33] that it is 'most likely a transient ischaemic attack involving temporal lobe structures'. Walton[34], states in *Brain's Diseases of the Nervous System* that TGA is 'believed to be due to transient ischaemia of one or both temporal lobes, as it usually occurs in middle aged or elderly individuals, with evidence of cerebral atherosclerosis'. A 1982 Leading Article in the *British Medical Journal*[35] states that 'increasingly the consensus has been that it has been due to vascular insufficiency affecting bilaterally the hypocampus'. Logan and Sherman[36], reviewing the topic in *Stroke*, conclude that, 'most authors feel that TGA represents a form of ischaemia on the basis on thrombo-embolic disease'.

Despite this overwhelming consensus there is little hard evidence to support a thromboembolic cause for TGA. The evidence marshalled in support is largely circumstantial or based on the analysis of risk factors for stroke (e.g. hypertension, ischaemic heart disease, diabetes, etc.) and long-term follow-up. Mathew and Meyer[37] performed the first systematic study of risk factors for stroke in their group of 14 patients. Since then a number of other authors have performed similar studies. These have resulted in an enormous variation in the estimated incidence of various risk factors[38–45]. These differences may depend, in part, upon definition of TGA, as when attacks accompanied by focal neurological features have been included within the rubric, the incidence of risk factors has tended to be high. A history of stroke occurred in 0–22% (average 4%), and of transient ischaemic attack (TIA) in 0–46% (average 14.5%). Accompanying hypertension was reported in 16–64% (average 38%). Ischaemic heart disease was present in 11–78% (average 30.5%) and diabetes mellitus in 1–28%. Two studies comment upon neck bruits, in 5% and 8% respectively. ECG abnormalities are reported in 9–44%.

Besides the problem with the inclusion criteria definition mentioned above, there are two major criticisms of all the studies reporting risk factors. First, *the method of data collection*. In all studies cases were ascertained retrospectively and the risk factor data collected from case record review. Any analysis based on such methodology must be viewed with scepticism. Secondly, *the lack of control data*. TGA occurs in the elderly, the mean age of cases in the reported larger series is 61 and in our series was 62 years. Many patients of this age will have incidental stroke risk factors and vascular abnormalities, purely by chance. To study relevant frequencies, cases must be compared with age- and sex-matched controls. There is only a small case control study, that of Kushner and Hauser[43]. They compared 18 cases to 90 age- and sex-matched hospital controls and found a very significant increase in risk factors, together with an extraordinarily high rate of previous stroke, in 12 of their 18 TGA patients (66%).

The present author's study was designed to address these methodological problems and to investigate the aetiology of TGA, by a series of case control studies. The prevalence of vascular risk factors in 114 well-defined and prospectively assessed cases of TGA was compared with two age- and sex-matched populations – first a group of 109 normal (community-based) controls and secondly a group of patients with conventional transient ischaemic attacks (TIAs) (see Figure 8.1). If the commonly held hypothesis

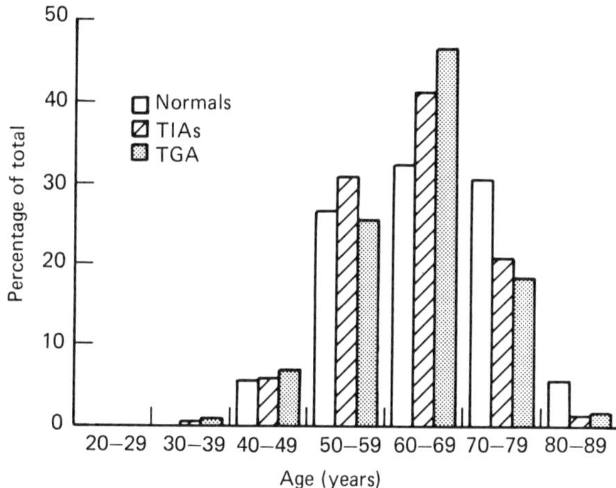

Figure 8.1 Age distribution of the case series and controls

that TGA represents a variety of thromboembolic cerebrovascular disease is correct, then there should be no difference in risk factors and outcome between TGA patients and those with conventional TIAs, but there may be significant differences in risk factors between TGA patients and normal controls. By contrast, if TGA is unrelated to cerebrovascular disease there should be significant differences in vascular risk factor prevalence and outcome between TGA and TIA cases and no difference between TGA and normal controls. In the author's study no significant differences were found in the prevalence of any vascular risk factors between TGAs and normal controls. Conversely, the following were significantly less common in TGAs than in TIA controls: hypertension, ischaemic and structural heart disease, carotid bruits, cigarette smoking and polycythaemia (see Table 8.2). We therefore found no evidence to support a cerebrovascular aetiology for TGA. Furthermore, long-term follow-up of the TGA and TIA groups showed a strikingly different prognosis. The rate of major vascular events adjusted for length of follow-up was 11 times greater in the TIA group (see Table 8.3)[46,47].

Table 8.2 Comparison of risk factors in TGA cases, normal controls and TIA controls

	TGA ($n = 114$)	Normal ($n = 109$)	TIA ($n = 212$)
Hypertension			
on treatment	17	26	32*
or systolic > 180 mmHg	37	36	51*
and/or diastolic > 100 mmHg			
Ischaemic heart disease	7	16	27*
Structural heart disease	7	14	17*
Atrial fibrillation (ECG proved)	3	–	3
Carotid bruits	9	9	30*
Peripheral vascular disease	4	2	15*
Polycythaemia (PCV > 50)	5	–	12*
Migraine			
any type	23†	11	14
classic	30†	17	20

Statistical comparison: 95% confidence interval of odds ratio > 1.0
* TIA > TGA
† TGA > normal and TIA

Table 8.3 Results of follow-up of TGA cases and TIA controls

	TGA ($n = 14$)	TIA ($n = 212$)	χ^2
Stroke	2	32	12.7‡
Myocardial infarct	0	16	7.5†
Death (total)	2	33	13.4‡
vascular causes	0	21	29.2‡
non-vascular causes	2	12	1.9
Stroke, myocardial infarct or vascular death	2	49	23.6‡

Mean follow-up: TGA, 34.8 months; TIA, 42.0 months
$P =$ *<0.05; †<0.01; ‡<0.001

The presence of CT scan abnormalities, particularly areas of infarction, has been used as evidence to support a cerebrovascular aetiology. Ladurner *et al.*[48] analysed the CT findings in 16 patients diagnosed as TGA. This material included three cases with fixed deficits (hemianopia, limb signs) and permanent memory loss. Not surprisingly all three with amnesic strokes had left posterior cerebral territory infarcts. Insufficient clinical details are provided in the other cases, four of whom had low density lesions. Very similar mixed series have been reported by other workers[41,44]. By contrast, Crowell[45] found no significant abnormalities in 12 patients undergoing CT scans. Caplan[31] reviewed the CT abnormalities in all reported cases and concluded that insufficient CT scan data were available to reach any general conclusions and that there is a need for a study of CT scan abnormalities in a larger group of patients with clearly defined TGA. CT scans were obtained in the majority of the present author's cases and no significant vascular lesions were found. It is no longer my practice to recommend routine CT scans in patients with typical TGA.

Epilepsy

Fisher and Adams[2] postulated that ischaemia of the ordinary cerebrovascular variety played no part and that most evidence was consistent with a form of cerebral seizure. A number of other authors also favour this mechanism[24,46–49]. The only compelling argument advanced in favour of epilepsy, by most authors, is the lack of another reasonable alternative diagnosis. Most reported cases of TGA are solitary and recurrence is unusual. Epilepsy is, by definition, a recurring condition, therefore patients with TGA cannot have what is usually meant by epilepsy. Conventional features of either generalized, or partial epilepsy are absent during the attack and the development of subsequent epilepsy is unusual. In addition, routine surface EEG recordings during and after TGA are normal or show minor non-specific abnormalities. Despite this evidence, several authors, have argued in favour of a form of cerebral seizure, localized to those structures subserving memory (the hippocampal-diencephalic system), as any abnormal discharges are likely to be deep within the brain and would not necessarily be accompanied by surface EEG abnormalities.

The EEG in TGA is a confusing and controversial topic. The early authors reported only minor post-attack abnormalities. In subsequent reports the proportion of abnormal EEGs after an attack varies from 0 to 60%. But most of the abnormalities consist of minor slow wave changes or excessive theta activity. A number of authors have reported single cases showing definite spike-and-wave discharges on inter-ictal recordings[46–49]. The specificity of these abnormalities has been challenged[50]. Other workers have found that nasopharyngeal lead recordings show spike discharges, even when routine EEG recordings were normal[48]. The comprehensive review of the EEG in TGA recently performed by Miller *et al.*[50], clarifies the situation considerably. They obtained EEG recordings during 13 episodes of TGA; 8 were entirely normal, none showed seizure activity. EEGs were also taken after episodes of TGA in 96 patients: more than 60% were normal, the remainder showed mild and non-specific focal abnormalities. The spectrum and the proportion of these abnormalities were similar to randomly selected and age-matched samples taken from the authors' files. My own experience is in keeping with this study.

The most important point remains that the vast majority of cases of TGA have normal conventional EEG recordings both during and after the attack. Of course, this is not to say that deeper limbic recordings may not show abnormality. All in all, evidence for conventional epilepsy as a cause for TGA is lacking. A minority of cases may develop epilepsy. In my own study 8 of the 114 patients have developed seizures, usually of temporal type and within one year of presentation. Most of these were initially after atypically brief and recurrent attacks.

Migraine

In addition to the two principal contenders – cerebrovascular disease and epilepsy – strong aetiological claims have been made recently for migraine. The occurrence of TGA in migraineurs was noted by several early authors[2,51,52]. More recently, Olivarius and Jensen[53] designated 'migrainous TGA' as a distinct sub-group with a benign outcome. Following up this suggestion, Caplan and co-workers[54] reported 12 selected cases from several centres in the United States of America and France, all with either a prior history of migraine or migraine accompaniments during TGA. Their cases were younger than is usual for TGA. The authors argue that many of the aspects of TGA, such as the precipitating factors, the predilection for the posterior circulation and the benign prognosis, could be explained by a migrainous aetiology.

Experimental support for the TGA/migraine connection comes from the study of Crowell and colleagues[45], who measured regional cerebral blood flow using a xenon-133 inhalation technique in seven patients at between 24 hours and 14 days after an attack. Five of those studied had abnormalities in the watershed area between the middle and posterior cerebral arteries and/or focal ischaemia in the inferior temporal lobe. This pattern of abnormalities is distinct from that seen after transient cerebral ischaemia. More recently, it has been suggested that the phenomenon of spreading depression (of Leao) might provide a unifying explanation for the cerebral blood flow abnormalities observed in migraine and for TGA[17,55].

Migrainous accompaniments, particularly headache, have been reported in a number of the larger series, with rates varying from 15% to 75%. It has been estimated that between 2% and 27% are migraineurs. In all these studies case ascertainment has been retrospective and the proportion with migraine presumably extracted from case note review. In our case-control study classic migraine was significantly more common in TGA cases than in either normal or TIA controls, occurring in 23%, 11% and 15% respectively.

Other

To add further to the confusion, individual case reports have claimed an association between TGA and a wide variety of other cerebral pathologies, including brain tumours, temporal lobe haemorrhage, subdural haematoma, drug toxicity, encephalitis, neurosyphilis, subarachnoid haemorrhage, aortic dissection, whiplash injury and covert head injury. However, when critically reviewed, most of these cases of so called 'symptomatic TGA' were either poorly witnessed or in some way atypical[31]. None of the author's 114 cases had such a cause.

Familial TGA

The first report of familial TGA was that of Corston and Godwin-Austen[22]. Their index case was a 63-year-old man who presented after two attacks. Three of his brothers had suffered similar episodes. This report stimulated a letter regarding a family with three affected members[56]. Recent reports have linked familial TGA with migraine in siblings with both conditions[57,58]. In the author's series of 114 cases two instances of 'familial TGA' were found, an overall prevalence of 1.8%. None of the other larger series has reported systematic studies of family history.

Natural history of TGA

The prognosis of TGA remains controversial. There have now been a number of follow-up studies of TGA patients, which have reached very different conclusions. Some have reported a very high rate of subsequent stroke whilst others have found no more than would be expected in a normal population of the same age. The major criticism of these studies is that none has included a control group of either normal subjects or patients with known cerebrovascular disease and none has analysed survival using actuarial methods.

The original authors felt that TGA was a benign syndrome with favourable outcome[2,3]. However, the first systematic follow-up study found a very high rate of stroke or vascular dementia[37,38]. Subsequently, others reported a very good outcome[38,41,59]. The findings in the only previous case-control follow-up by Kushner and Hauser[43], were contradictory, in that although 12 of their 18 patients had suffered prior cerebral ischaemia, none had subsequent strokes on follow-up. A Danish group[44] were the first to compare outcome in their patients with a known population stroke rate. They obtained 100% follow-up in 74 well-defined cases. In 415 patient-years of follow-up there are only three strokes, which was no more than the estimated rate. More recently, a study from the Mayo Clinic of 277 patients seen over a 15 year period reached a similar conclusion. Only 11 patients had subsequent strokes and the calculated incidence (595 per 100 000 patient-years) was no higher than expected[50].

The long-term follow-up of my own series of 114 patients confirms an excellent prognosis. Only two have died (in more than 300 patient-years of follow-up), both of non-vascular causes, and two had cerebrovascular accidents, a rate of 613 per 100 000 patient-years. The incidence of major vascular events was no higher than expected for that age group but was significantly less than the matched TIA control group.

Recurrence rate

The apparently low recurrence rate has been one of the most difficult facts to accommodate in any aetiological theory. Most authors stressed the singleness of TGA. However, a review of the literature reveals recurrence rates from 6% to 57%; the higher rates tend to be those of the earlier studies[24,37,41] in which diagnostic criteria were not clearly stated and cases with additional neurological features were included. When more stringent criteria have been applied recurrence rates are much lower[38,39,43]. The only studies to take duration of follow-up into account are those by Hinge *et al.*[42], who found an average annual recurrence rate of 4.7% and the author's own, with a 3% annual recurrence rate.

Conclusions

TGA is probably much more common than is recognized as we have been able to study more than 100 cases locally. It is a highly characteristic clinical syndrome. Much of the confusion in the literature regarding the aetiology of TGA results from inconsistencies in the use of the diagnostic term. I have suggested firm criteria for the diagnosis. Most authors accept that cerebrovascular disease of the thromboembolic type is the cause of TGA. However, the supporting evidence is largely circumstantial. Our case control studies provide no support for this as a cause. Patients fulfilling the proposed criteria have an excellent prognosis and can be reassured by the low recurrence rate. Evidence for epilepsy is largely lacking. A small proportion of cases may eventually develop epilepsy. The EEG is normal or shows minimal non-specific abnormalities, both during and after TGA. Migraine does appear to be associated with TGA and this area warrants further investigation.

References

1. FISHER, C. M. and ADAMS, R. D. *Trans. Am. Neurol. Assoc.*, **83**, 143 (1958)
2. FISHER, C. M. and ADAMS, R. D. *Acta Neurol. Scand.*, **40** (Suppl. 9), 1 (1964)
3. BENDER, M. B. *J. Hillside Hosp.*, **5**, 212 (1956)
4. BENDER, M. B. *Bull. NY Acad. Med.*, **36**, 197 (1960)
5. GUYOTAT, J. and COURJON, J. *J. Med. Lyon*, **37**, 697 (1956)
6. JEQUIER, M. *et al. Rev. Med.*, **89**, 697 (1969)
7. FAU, R., GARREL, S., GROSLAMBERT, R. *et al. Semin. Hôp. Paris*, **46**, 1275 (1970)
8. HAAS, D. C. *Arch. Neurol. (Chicago)*, **40**, 258 (1983)
9. KANZER, M. *Am. J. Psych.*, **96**, 711 (1939)
10. CAFFARRA, P., MORETTI, G., MAZZUCCHI, A. and PARMA, M. *Acta Neurol. Scand.*, **63**, 44 (1981)
11. HODGES, J. R., WARD, C. D., OSTERGAARD, A. *et al. Brain* (in press)
12. REGARD, M. and LANDIS, T. *J. Neurol. Neurosurg. Psychiat.*, **47**, 668 (1984)
13. SQUIRE, L. R. *Science*, **232**, 1612 (1986)
14. PARKIN, A. J. *Cortex*, **20**, 479 (1984)
15. MILNER, B. *Br. Med. Bull.*, **27**, 272 (1971)
16. CASTAIGNE, P., LHERMITTE, F., BUGE, A. *et al. Ann. Neurol.*, **10**, 127 (1981)
17. LAURITZEN, M. D., OLSEN, T. S., LASSEN, N. A. *et al. Ann. Neurol.*, **13**, 633 (1983)
18. MARTIN, E. A. *Irish J. Med. Sci.*, **3**, 331 (1970)
19. FISHER, C. M. *Arch. Neurol.*, **39**, 605 (1982)
20. VAN CREVEL, H. *J. Psychiat. Neurol. Neurochir.*, **72**, 319 (1969)
21. MAYEUX, R. *N. Engl. J. Med.*, **300**, 364 (1979)
22. CORSTON, R. N. and GODWIN-AUSTEN, R. B. *J. Neurol. Neurosurg. Psychiat.*, **45**, 375 (1982)
23. HEATHFIELD, K. W. G., CROFT, P. B. and SWASH, M. *Brain*, **96**, 729 (1973)
24. GODLEWSKI, S. *Semin. Hôp. Paris*, **44**, 553 (1968)
25. BOLWIG, T. G. *Acta Neurol. Scand.*, **44**, 101 (1968)
26. MAN-SON-HING, C. T. *Can. Med. Assoc. J.*, **98**, 594 (1968)
27. WALES, L. R. and NOV, A. A. *Am. J. Neuroradiol. (Baltimore)*, **2**, 275 (1981)
28. COCHRAN, J. W., MORRELL, F., HUCKMAN, M. S. and COCHRAN, E. J. *Arch. Neurol. (Chicago)*, **39**, 593 (1982)
29. PEXMAN, J. H. W. and COATES, R. K. *J. Neuroradiol. (Baltimore)*, **4**, 979 (1983)
30. SHUTTLEWORTH, E. C. and WISE, G. R. *Arch. Neurol.*, **29**, 340 (1973)

31. CAPLAN, L. R. In *Handbook of Clinical Neurology* (ed. P. J. Vinken, G. W. Bruyn and H. L. Klawans), Elsevier Science, London, vol. 1, p. 205 (1985)
32. HAAS, D. C. and ROSS, G. S. *Brain,* **109**, 251 (1986)
33. ADAMS, R. D. and VICTOR, M. *Principles of Neurology,* 3rd edn, McGraw-Hill, New York, 319 (1985)
34. WALTON, J. *Brain's Diseases of the Nervous System,* 9th edn, Oxford University Press, Oxford, p. 653 (1985)
35. LEADING ARTICLE. *Br. Med. J.,* **4**, 723 (1968)
36. LOGAN, W. and SHERMAN, D. G. *Stroke,* **14**, 1005 (1983)
37. MATHEW, N. T. and MEYER, J. S. *Stroke,* **5**, 303 (1974)
38. NAUSIEDA, P. A. and SHERMAN, I. C. *JAMA,* **241**, 392 (1979)
39. SHUPING, J. R. and TOOLE, J. F. *Ann. Neurol.,* **7**, 281 (1980)
40. JENSEN, T. S. and OLIVARIUS, B. de F. *Arch. Neurol. Scand.,* **63**, 220 (1981)
41. CATTAINO, G., QUERIN, F., POMES, A. and PIAZZA, P. *Acta Neurol. Scand.,* **70**, 385 (1984)
42. HINGE, H. H., JENSEN, T. S., KJAER, M. *et al. Arch. Neurol.,* **43**, 673 (1986)
43. KUSHNER, M. J. and HAUSER, W. A. *Ann. Neurol.,* **18**, 684 (1985)
44. MATIAS-GUIU, J., COLOMER, R., SEGURA, A. and CODINA, A. *Acta Neurol. Scand.,* **73**, 298 (1986)
45. CROWELL, G. F., STUMP, D. A., BILLER, J. *et al. Arch. Neurol.,* **41**, 75 (1984)
46. THARP, B. R. *Electroencephalogr. Clin. Neurophysiol.,* **26**, 96 (1969)
47. LOU, H. O. C. *Acta Neurol. Scand.,* **44**, 612 (1968)
48. LADURNER, G., SKVARC, A. and SAGER, W. D. *Eur. Neurol.,* **21**, 34 (1982)
49. STEINMETZ, E. F. and VROOM, F. Q. *Neurology,* **22**, 1193 (1972)
50. MILLER, J. W., YANAGIHARA, T., PETERSEN, R. C. and KLASS, D. W. *Arch. Neurol.,* **44**, 629 (1987)
51. EVANS, J. H. *Brain,* **89**, 539 (1966)
52. GILBERT, J. J. and BENSON, D. F. *J. Nerv. Ment. Dis.,* **154**, 461 (1972)
53. OLIVARIUS, B. de F. and JENSEN, T. S. *Headache,* **19**, 335 (1979)
54. CAPLAN, L. R., CHEDRU, F., LHERMITTE, F. and MAYMAN, C. *Neurology,* **31**, 1167 (1981)
55. OLESEN, J. and JORGENSEN, M. B. *Acta Neurol. Scand.,* **73**, 219 (1986)
56. MUNRO, J. M. and LOIZOU, L. A. *J. Neurol. Neurosurg. Psychiat.,* **45**, 1070 (1982)
57. STRACCIARI, A. and REBUCCI, G. G. *J. Neurol. Neurosurg. Psychiat.,* **49**, 716 (1986)
58. DUPUIS, M. J. M., PIERRE, P. H. and GONSETTE, R. E. *J. Neurol. Neurosurg. Psychiat.,* **50**, 816 (1987)
59. FOGELHOLM, R., KIVALO, E. and BERGSTROM, L. *Eur. Neurol.,* **13**, 72 (1975)

Chapter 9

Ageing and the response to injury

M. A. Horan, R. N. Barton and R. A. Little

Introduction

Why are responses to injury within the context of ageing a valid area for scientific investigation? One reason is that large numbers of old people sustain injuries as a result of surgical procedures as well as accidentally, and age-related changes in injury responses may influence morbidity and fatality. A further reason is that more fundamental issues may be addressed regarding the functional significance of the numerous age-related changes described in many systems. Over the past few decades, the major thrust in ageing research has been to describe the influence of ageing on very well-defined functions such as the activity of a particular enzyme or the functioning of a particular cell type, usually under basal conditions. Most gerontologists have not gone on to define the functional significance of such changes within the system in which they were designed to operate. This is especially surprising since ageing has often been considered philosophically within the context of homeostasis and deviations in homeostasis[1]. It is probably true to say that most age-related changes are in themselves relatively minor, but their presence within complex, integrated systems in the intact organism may have effects out of all proportion to what is seen in the original experimental system.

It is widely held that elderly people are more vulnerable to the effects of injury than their younger counterparts. Even though people over the age of 65 account for only 25% of all surgical admissions, they account for around 75% of postoperative deaths[2]. Postoperative morbidity is also higher in this group, as is evidenced by the considerably longer duration of hospital stay[2].

The incidence of accidental injuries in people over the age of 65 is relatively low, but this belies their importance since old people who sustain such injuries are much more likely to die as a result[3–5]. When *deaths* from injury are plotted against age, there is a small peak in the 15–24 age group and a much larger peak in the age group 75–84 years. This general pattern is true at all anatomical sites (e.g. head, trunk, limbs) and was shown to be very similar when the decades 1947–1956 and 1962–1971 were compared[3]. When these figures are further analysed, it is clear that fractures of the upper femur account for most of the peak in old age.

It has been reported that at ages of 65 and above fractures of the upper femur affect 2.3 per 1000 men and 6.0 per 1000 women annually and the incidence rises markedly with advancing age[6,7]. It is believed that demographic changes over the next two decades will result in an increase in the number of patients with fractures of the upper femur by a factor of 2.7. Indeed, a rising incidence of fracture of the femoral neck has already been recorded[7–14]. The study by Hedlund, Ahlbom and Lindgren[13] showed a relatively greater rise in the incidence of intertrochanteric over subcapital and transcervical fractures. Boyce and Vessey[14] suggest that new risk factors may have emerged or old risk factors may be of increasing frequency and/or severity.

It is generally believed that age-related bone loss (osteoporosis) is the most important risk factor for fractures of the upper femur. Melton and co-workers[15] have recently quantified the influence of bone density (and presumably bone strength) on the risk of hip fractures. Fractures were very rare in women with a femoral bone density of $1.0\,\mathrm{g/cm^2}$ but the incidence was 8.3 per 1000 person-years with a cervical bone density of less than $0.6\,\mathrm{g/cm^2}$ and 16.6 per 1000 person-years with an intertrochanteric bone density of less than $0.6\,\mathrm{g/cm^2}$.

Observations such as these should alert us to the possible dangers of comparing injuries between different age groups. For example, the force required to fracture the femur will be considerably less in an old person with thin bones than in a young person with a greater bone mass, and the associated soft tissue injury is likely to be less extensive. However, injury severity will be determined not only by the amount of tissue damage but also by the loss of fluid from the circulation. The ability to compensate for this circulatory hypovolaemia will be compromised if autonomic nervous system function is impaired. The sensitivity of the baroreflex in man declines with increasing age[16,17] and there is evidence for central impairment of baroreflex control of vasopressin secretion in the elderly[18]. Peripheral vasoconstriction may also be compromised by a decrease in sensitivity to noradrenaline that is released[19]. The preservation of blood flow to vital organs after injury will be determined by compensation for circulatory hypovolaemia and by the efficiency of autoregulation of local blood flow. Cerebral blood flow appears to be well maintained in old age, unless pathological conditions are superimposed[20,21]; however there are differences in the ability of young and old rats to autoregulate cortical blood flow in response to hypercapnia[22].

Several systems for assessing the severity of injury have been suggested. Most have been developed from data in younger people and they cannot be applied indiscriminately to the elderly. For anatomically based systems the factors discussed above will have opposing effects: osteoporosis will tend to cause injury severity to be overestimated in old people whereas impaired compensation will do the opposite. As far as mortality is concerned the latter effect seems to predominate; for the most commonly used system, the Injury Severity Score (ISS)[23], the LD_{50} decreases with age[4]. However, this is probably not related solely to the acute effects of injury, as the proportion of deaths that occur more than one day later is greater for patients aged over 65 than for younger ones[4]. The relationships between acute metabolic changes and ISS do not seem to change with age in the same way as those for survival[4], as will be discussed below. In physiologically based injury-scoring systems, such as the Trauma Score[24] and APACHE II[25], the age-related changes in tissue damage and compensation will be reflected to some extent in the variables these systems include, but some authors consider it necessary to introduce an additional weighting for age. This seems largely speculative and again may not be equally appropriate for all applications of the scales. Thus, in the APACHE II system a weighting for age is recommended only if mortality is being studied[25].

Late deaths occur in elderly people after injuries of a severity that would cause few younger patients to die. Femoral neck fracture carries a substantial mortality in the elderly and the peak death rate is one month after injury[3]. The death rate continues at an increased level for a considerable time, reported as 12 months by one group[26] and 20 months by another[27]. The reasons for this remain a mystery. Comprehensive post-mortem studies have not been done and attributing death to pneumonia, pulmonary embolism and so forth may be misleading.

In this review we consider the effects of ageing on the general response to injury, concentrating on heat production and thermo-regulation, the neuroendocrine and metabolic changes and the activity of the reticuloendothelial system. Within these areas we have tried to give a comprehensive account of the literature, but as this is sparse, we have sometimes had to confine ourselves to predictions based on age-associated changes in uninjured indi-viduals. We have taken 'elderly' to mean over 65 years of age, but it is likely that very old patients, who are frequently victims of femoral neck fracture, will show differences from those in their sixties and early seventies. Conversely, much of the literature on 'normal' responses to elective surgery is based on patients aged over 50, and sharp differences from moderately elderly patients should perhaps not be expected.

Heat production and thermoregulation

Metabolic rate (or heat production) is a major factor in the control of body temperature. Metabolic rate is most often calculated by the method of indirect calorimetry, which involves the measurement of whole body oxygen consumption and, ideally, carbon dioxide production[28]. Oxygen consumption normally has two components. There is a basal part, which maintains heart, lung and central nervous system functions and ionic gradients in a post-absorptive, resting state in a thermoneutral environment[29]. In addition, there is a thermoregulatory or external energy expenditure at temperatures outside the thermoneutral zone.

When considering any aspect of the metabolic response to injury it is both conventional and convenient to use the terminology introduced by Cuthbertson in 1942[30]. Immediately after injury there is the 'ebb' phase, so called because it was thought to be characterized by a reduction in metabolic rate. In patients who do not die acutely, this is followed by the 'flow' phase of enhanced metabolic activity. As there are no data for the elderly on these aspects of the response to accidental injury, the discussion that follows will be restricted to the responses described for young adult experimental animals and humans. We shall then consider the physiological changes associated with ageing that might be expected to modify these responses and briefly discuss some of the few relevant studies of elderly patients undergoing elective surgery.

The ebb phase

The most complete description of the changes in metabolic rate in this phase comes from studies in experimental animals. At environmental temperatures below the thermoneutral zone oxygen consumption is reduced after injury and the magnitude of the reduction, at a given environmental temperature, is directly related to the severity of injury[31]. The reduction in oxygen consumption is due not to failure of tissue oxygen transport but to central inhibition of thermoregulation. Both nociceptive impulses arising from damaged tissues and fluid loss from the circulation contribute to this phenomenon. The effects of nociceptive impulses appear to be mediated by neurones whose axons ascend to the region of the dorsomedial nucleus of the hypothalamus where they release noradrenaline. These neural changes lead to inhibition of shivering thermogenesis and a reduction in the ambient and hypothalamic temperature thresholds for increasing heat production[32,33]. The superimposition of fluid loss from the circulation on to the changes produced by tissue injury leads to a further lowering of the ambient and hypothalamic thresholds for shivering and to inhibition of non-shivering thermogenesis in liver and brown adipose tissue. Body temperature and whole-body oxygen consumption fall at ambient temperatures below the zone of thermoneutrality; however, oxygen consumption does not fall below basal and only the thermoregulatory component of heat production is inhibited[34].

The evidence for inhibition of thermoregulatory heat production in man after injury is not nearly so clear. The median metabolic rate measured by indirect calorimetry shortly after accidental injury was similar to that in control subjects under similar environmental conditions[35,36]. However, the metabolic rate was significantly more variable in the injured and, in some patients, values as low as 50% of predicted were recorded; such low values appeared to be most common in the elderly although there were too few to test statistically. The physiological significance of this finding is difficult to decide because the emergency room is often at a temperature close to the thermoneutral zone so that thermoregulatory heat production is low.

There is no doubt that core temperature is reduced in man shortly after severe injury and that the reduction is directly related to the severity of the injury[37]. The mechanism of this fall in temperature is not known but it is a feature of such patients that they do not shiver despite having body temperatures below the normal threshold for the onset of shivering. This may be secondary to the reduction in arterial baroreceptor input to the brain[38], but it is tempting to speculate that it is due rather to central inhibition of thermoregulation. There is indeed some evidence of inhibition of both behavioural and autonomic thermoregulatory reflexes at this time after injury[39]. The selection of an 'ambient' temperature that maximizes thermal comfort is an accepted test of behavioural thermoregulation. In control subjects a pleasurable temperature for the hand depends on core temperature to which it is negatively related. This normal negative relationship between preferred hand ambient temperature and core temperature is lost shortly after accidental injury.

The flow phase

There is no doubt that in experimental animals and in man metabolic rate is increased in the flow phase of the response to both thermal and non-thermal injuries and the extent of the hypermetabolism is directly related to the severity of injury. Multiple long-bone fractures increase metabolic rate by some 10–20%, to 1500–2000 kcal/day, for 1–2 weeks after injury[40], but metabolic rate can increase above 3500 kcal/day after major burns[41] and also, intermittently, after major head injuries[42]. It seems that a doubling of metabolic rate is the maximal response that can be maintained for any length of time owing to the limitations imposed by the cardiovascular and respiratory systems. In patients with multiple injuries there are a number of reasons why metabolic rates above 1500–2000 kcal/day are not usually seen: for example, food intake may be limited acutely after injury owing to anorexia and physical activity is reduced because of immobilization. All these factors reduce metabolic rate with the result that the hypermetabolic flow phase response is superimposed on a declining background of resting energy expenditure.

The pathogenesis of the hypermetabolism in the flow phase is not completely understood and a number of factors may contribute[43]. For example, there may be a central upward resetting of thermoregulation[28,44] and the wound may be acting as an additional organ[45–47]. The wound may increase metabolic rate not only because of the high oxygen consumption of its tissues but also through the increased heart work required to maintain its blood flow and the metabolic work involved in converting the lactate it produces to glucose in the liver. The increased protein synthesis and breakdown associated with the flow phase also have an energy cost and after burning injury the latent heat of evaporation from the wound surface has to be provided.

Metabolic rate and thermoregulation in the elderly

The changes in metabolic rate after injury will be influenced by the pre-existing metabolic rate. A reduction in metabolic rate with increasing age is well recognized[48,49]. Although thyroid hormone secretion also decreases with age, this does not seem to be responsible[50]. The fall in metabolic rate is best explained by an age-related decrease in skeletal muscle and metabolic mass[51]. This decrease in muscle cell mass is associated with a fall in the rate of muscle protein turnover[52], an energy-consuming process.

Metabolic rate is also influenced by calorie intake and activity. The decrease in cell mass in the elderly will be accompanied by a reduction in calorie intake. This reduction will be exacerbated by anorexia in patients with gastric disease, the prevalence of which increases with age. Physical activity is reduced in the elderly and it has been shown that the calorie expenditure for activity falls somewhat more than that for basal metabolism[53].

The control of metabolic rate is intimately associated with that of thermoregulation (see above) and there is substantial evidence that the ability to thermoregulate is adversely affected during ageing in both experimental animals[54–59] and man. The elderly have a reduced ability to discriminate differences in environmental temperature and a lack of precision in manipulating their thermal environment to achieve comfort[60,61]. There are also age-related impairments in the regulation of both heat loss and heat production. The ability to reduce heat loss is compromised and this has been associated with a failure of autonomic regulation of peripheral blood flow[62,63]. Shivering is less pronounced in the elderly on exposure to cold[64] and this may be due, in part, to a reduction in muscle mass and power. The amount of brown adipose tissue decreases throughout life and although it can be reactivated by cold exposure in the elderly its quantitative importance in thermogenesis remains controversial[65]. There is evidence that the thermogenic response of brown adipose tissue to cold is markedly reduced in the aged rat[66] and it has recently been suggested that this could be mediated in some way by the hypothalamus–pituitary–adrenal axis as the effects of age can be reversed by adrenalectomy[67] and corticotrophin-releasing factor may be involved in the stimulation of brown fat[68]. There is no evidence to suggest a lack of substrate availability for thermogenesis in the elderly during the ebb phase (see pp. 117–120, below).

Thermoregulation, like metabolic rate, can be impaired by deficiencies in food intake. A 20 hour fast or an isocaloric protein-restricted diet limits the ability of mice to maintain body temperature on cold exposure[69,70]. Elderly undernourished patients when compared with normally nourished controls have a reduced increase in metabolic rate on cold exposure which is associated with a fall (rather than the expected rise) in plasma catecholamine concentrations[71]. It has been proposed that, in the severely undernourished elderly subject in cold weather, the drop in body temperature is such as to cause incoordination leading to a fall and possibly injury (e.g. fractured neck of femur). There may well be further impairment of thermoregulation after injury and as a result these patients are hypothermic on admission to hospital[72]. The development of hypothermia can be very rapid; all the patients in this study were examined within 4 hours of injury, which is consistent with the calculation that even without injury an elderly person who does not shiver can become hypothermic after only 5 hours of cold exposure[73].

As mentioned above, the magnitude of an increase in metabolic rate after injury can be limited by constraints imposed by the cardiovascular and respiratory systems. The maintenance of cardiac output is impaired with increasing age[74]. This may be associated with the increasing infiltration of the myocardium with collagen[75] as the elderly rely more on a change in stroke volume than in heart rate to increase cardiac output[53]. There are also changes in pulmonary function with age such that vital capacity and maximal breathing capacity are reduced[76]. The rigidity of the rib cage increases with age, which means that the diaphragm becomes more important in gas exchange; however, the function of the diaphragm can be adversely affected by malnutrition and by abdominal surgery. Oxygen uptake in the lung may also be impaired in the elderly[77]. These changes in cardiovascular and pulmonary function mean that the maximal capacity for tissue oxygen delivery[78], and hence the ability to maintain a hyper-metabolic state, might be expected to decline with age. In this respect the response to injury would be a good example of how the need for the integrated activity of a number of homeostatic systems most exposes the deleterious effects of ageing on the individual systems[79].

The influence of these many age-related changes does not appear to have been analysed experimentally in elderly patients after accidental injury. The most comprehensive study of thermo-regulation after trauma in old people is probably that of Renck[80], who studied the responses to prostatectomy in men aged 60–86. Oxygen consumption appeared to be greater than expected during the first 24 hours after operation, although no data for younger subjects were included. The oldest patients had the lowest Po_2 values, the most difficulty in normalizing body temperature and the greatest decreases in physical working capacity. The author emphasized the desirability of minimizing postoperative oxygen consumption by preventing blood loss and pain, and suggested active rewarming as a therapeutic measure. In a series reported in 1986 Carli and Itiaba[81] tried rewarming elderly patients undergoing lower abdominal surgery and found it to have a beneficial effect in reducing the net protein catabolic response to the injury.

Neuroendocrine response

Rapid increases in the secretion of many hormones occur as a result of several types of stimulus produced by injury. These may originate in the special senses and higher centres, from tissue damage (via nociceptive afferents ascending in the spinal cord) and from fluid loss, with a lessening of the inhibitory neural input from low- and high-pressure baroreceptors[82,83]. These ebb phase responses subside at rates depending upon the hormone and the severity of injury, so that hormone concentrations may return to normal within a few hours or still be elevated well into the flow phase. For some hormones, especially insulin, the thyroid hormones and the gonadal steroids, this phase produces its own characteristic disturbances in regulation[83].

Apart from the hypothalamus–pituitary–adrenal axis, little is known of the effects of ageing on these responses, and it is difficult to predict what might be expected. Most work on the endocrine effects of ageing has been on basal hormone levels and the effects of physiological stimuli. It is clear from the many reviews of this work that there is no common pattern of change, and in fact for many hormones it is remarkable how little change with age there appears to be. Davis[84] has identified three recurring features: primary changes in secretion, decreased rates of degradation and alterations in end organ sensitivity. (Gregerman[85] has widened these categories even further.) Of these, one might expect the second to have the most predictable effect on the neuroendocrine response, in leading to higher concentrations of the hormones concerned. Changes in end organ sensitivity might well affect secondary hormone responses and particularly (through changes in feedback inhibition) the rate at which the neuroendocrine response subsides. It is also possible that ageing affects the stimuli elicited by injury and the pathways by which information is transferred to the neuroendocrine regulatory centres (hypothalamus and medullary sympathetic area) in the brain. For example, it has been suggested that arteriosclerosis leads to a reduction in carotid baroreceptor tone[86] and decreased sensitivity to hypotension might be expected. However, there is so far no evidence that this has a substantial effect on the neuroendocrine response to injury. Changes in central neurotransmitters with age have also been reported[87] but their implications for the neuroendocrine response are not clear.

Hypothalamus–pituitary–adrenal axis

Before discussing the effects of injury, it will be helpful to summarize the large amount of work that has been done on the normal effects of ageing. The only change on which there is general agreement[84] is that cortisol clearance decreases[88], although Serio *et al.*[89] found that even this was not statistically significant. One would therefore expect that, after adrenocortico-trophic hormone (ACTH) administration, the peak plasma cortisol concentration (though not the initial rise) would be greater in the old than in the young. Although Friedman *et al.*[90] found that this was so, most other workers have found unchanged plasma cortisol responses to even prolonged ACTH infusions[88,91], and this led West *et al.*[88] to postulate that the maximal secretory response to ACTH decreases similarly in old age. This is supported by the finding of a lower urinary excretion of 17-hydroxycorticosteroids, a rough indicator of cortisol production rate[92]. Under basal conditions most workers find that the plasma concentrations of cortisol[88,93–95] (but see[90]) and ACTH[93,95,96] are unchanged in old age. This suggests that cortisol secretion in response to physiological concentrations of ACTH is also decreased and that feedback inhibition of the hypothalamus–pituitary–adrenal (HPA) axis by cortisol is intact. There is evidence for both propositions. The cortisol production rate[97] and the urinary excretion of 17-ketogenic steroids[93] decrease with age, whereas dexamethasone suppresses the HPA axis normally[90,94]. There is so far no evidence that the impairment of feedback inhibition observed in aged animals, and attributed to loss of glucocorticoid receptors in the hippocampus[98], occurs with normal ageing in man. However, suppressibility by dexamethasone does not necessarily imply normal feedback inhibition by physiological cortisol concentrations.

Most studies of the effects of trauma on the HPA axis in the elderly have used elective surgery as the trauma. Early workers[99,100] showed that the increased susceptibility of the elderly to surgical trauma was not due to failure to mount an adrenocortical response. Subsequently, in more detailed studies, Blichert-Toft[93] showed that the initial rise in plasma cortisol was similar in elderly (age 65–84) and younger (age 17–60) patients undergoing major surgery. However, during the first few hours after surgery plasma cortisol was higher and more variable in the elderly, and it continued to be higher for the next four days provided samples were taken in the evening; apparently morning samples did not give such a clear picture. Age had no effect on urinary 17-ketogenic steroid excretion during this period, although it was higher (and more variable) in the elderly if expressed as a percentage increase over basal. Plasma cortisol was also higher in old than in young patients during the first few hours after more minor surgery[101]. There was no difference in ACTH between age groups either 1 hour or 5 days after major surgery[102].

These data clearly confirm that the adrenal cortex responds adequately to elective surgery in the elderly, but further interpretation is difficult. The finding of higher plasma cortisol levels without (in absolute terms) correspondingly raised 17-ketogenic steroid excretion would be consistent with the decreased cortisol clearance found in normal old people, provided the same proportion of cortisol was converted to these metabolites. The old people's higher plasma cortisol but similar ACTH 1 hour after surgery might suggest that this decreased clearance was no longer offset by a diminished response of the adrenal cortex to ACTH; however, the two hormones were not determined in the same patients. An effect of surgery on adrenocortical responsiveness in the elderly was also suggested by the results of tests with metyrapone, which inhibits the conversion of 11-deoxycortisol to cortisol and thus abolishes tonic feedback inhibition of the HPA axis. Before surgery the rise in plasma 11-deoxycortisol was similar in the young and old patients, whereas 5–6 days after surgery it was higher in the old[93]. (Urinary 17-ketogenic steroid excretion rose similarly in the two postoperative groups; it was apparently not measured in the preoperative test.) However, interpretation of these data is difficult because of uncertainties over whether the increase in ACTH was similar in the two age groups. Although it probably was preoperatively[96], the postoperative rise could have been greater in the aged as many values were off-scale[102].

Other studies of the adrenocortical response to surgery in the elderly do not add much to these findings. Querido and van Seters[103] showed that the cortisol secretion rate increased, and Bowen and Richardson[104] and Oyama *et al.*[105] found perhaps greater than expected rises in plasma cortisol, but none of these studies included younger groups for comparison. Håkanson *et al.*[106] did study two groups, but as the ages were not well separated (<55 and >55, with a maximum age of 71), it is perhaps not surprising that they found no difference in the plasma cortisol response to cholecystectomy.

We and our colleagues have studied the HPA axis in elderly patients with accidental injuries. Within the first few hours of receiving injuries that were comparable by the ISS[23], plasma cortisol and ACTH were raised similarly in elderly and younger patients[107,108]. However, in the group with most homogeneous injuries (ISS 9–11, with the major injury in the lower limbs – in the elderly these were mostly fractures of the femoral neck), cortisol was significantly more variable in the elderly; a similar comparison could not be made of ACTH because of its non-normal statistical distribution[108]. Systematic follow-up studies were not done until 1 week after injury, when elderly patients with a fracture of the neck of the femur had higher cortisol concentrations than younger patients even with greater ISS values; the difference persisted for at least another 1–2 weeks[109]. These findings are consistent with those of Blichert-Toft[93] after elective surgery.

Why an elevated cortisol concentration should be so persistent in elderly patients with a fracture of the femoral neck is unclear. Frayn *et al.*[109] found similarly high cortisol concentrations in inactive elderly control subjects, in contrast to active ones, and suggested that immobility rather than injury *per se* was responsible. As the plasma insulin concentration was also raised, a possible explanation was a decrease in liver blood flow with consequent impairment of cortisol clearance. Measurement of plasma ACTH seemed to confirm this, for in patients 1–3 weeks after femoral neck fracture it was at the lower end of the normal range, as might be expected if feedback inhibition by cortisol were occurring[110]. However, administration of $[^3H]$cortisol to such patients has shown that their cortisol production rate is similar to that in younger control subjects and thus higher than normal for their age (77–88), so that undue impairment of cortisol clearance does not seem to be the whole explanation[110]. Increased binding of cortisol to plasma proteins is not involved, for free cortisol increases commensurately with the total cortisol concentration in plasma[110].

We do not yet have an explanation for this apparent discrepancy between cortisol secretion rate and plasma ACTH and are currently performing simple tests of adrenal function in patients at different stages after femoral neck fracture to try to characterize the disturbances more fully. In the meantime two points are worth making. First, at no stage after accidental injury are relationships between cortisol and ACTH straightforward[83]; even within the first two hours there is no clear correlation between the two hormone concentrations[108]. Second, it is now clear that immobility does not consistently increase plasma cortisol. Vernikos[111] concludes that, on the contrary, immobility usually reduces sensitivity to stimulation by ACTH. However, in contrast to most other workers, she finds a similar effect of ageing (55–65 v. 25–35 years), which she attributes to decreased activity. In addition, she presents data that appear to show an increase in plasma cortisol without a corresponding rise in ACTH during the first 20 days of bed-rest, although this is not commented on.

Other pituitary hormones

In younger patients, the early neuroendocrine response to injury includes rises in the concentrations of growth hormone (GH), prolactin and vasopressin, with no consistent change in thyroid-stimulating hormone (TSH) or the gonadotrophins[82,83]. Of these, only GH appears to have been studied after trauma in the elderly. Blichert-Toft[93] showed that during the first few hours after major surgery plasma GH was lower in elderly than in younger patients despite higher preoperative levels in the former. There were no consistent differences between the age groups during the next four days, or in the response to intravenous arginine at the end of this period. Measurement of cortisol in the same patients showed that the lower postoperative GH levels did not represent a general decrease in anterior pituitary response, and the reason for them is not clear. Most studies of GH in the elderly have shown unchanged basal levels and responses to stimuli such as insulin-induced hypoglycaemia, and the abnormality most frequently reported is a decrease in the number of spontaneous episodes of secretion[112]. The effect of ageing on the responses of other pituitary hormones to injury is difficult to predict. In normal individuals ageing causes little change in the basal concentrations of prolactin or TSH, and an increase in those of the gonadotrophins, but the effects of stress do not appear to have been studied[50,84]. Rowe *et al.*[18] have shown that the rise in vasopressin on standing is decreased in old age. This suggests that ageing could reduce the vasopressin response to those injuries in which hypovolaemia is an important stimulus, as opposed to elective surgery where vasopressin release is largely due to nociception[113].

During the flow phase after injury in younger subjects there are disturbances in the regulation of thyroid and sex hormones, the main manifestations of which are a fall in the concentrations of triiodothyronine(T_3) and, in males, testosterone, without corresponding changes in TSH or gonadotrophins (the changes in females have been poorly characterized)[83]. These appear to be general effects of illness rather than specific effects of injury. There is a tendency for both changes to be seen in elderly populations and Davis[84] and Gregerman and Bierman[50] have concluded that this is largely due to inclusion of unhealthy individuals. This presupposes that illness will have the same effects in the elderly, and thus it seems highly likely that in them both T_3 and, in males, testosterone will decrease a few days after injury. Blichert-Toft *et al.*[101] found that inguinal herniorrhaphy caused a fall in serum T_3 in elderly males, similar to that in young ones, but as this started before skin incision it is unlikely to have been the same phenomenon; patients were not followed beyond 6 hours afterwards. As regards other hormones, changes with ageing in the normal regulatory mechanisms could well come into play during the flow phase, e.g. the increase in sensitivity of vasopressin secretion to osmolality reported with ageing[50,84], but again there is little specific information.

Sympatho-adrenal system

Despite its crucial role in the response to injury, most studies of the sympatho-adrenal system in old people have used only minor stimuli (standing, isometric exercise etc.) and have measured only noradrenaline and not adrenaline, which is physiologically easier to interpret and is regulated very differently[114]. The usual finding is that resting plasma noradrenaline increases with age, perhaps because of decreased carotid baroreceptor tone, and so does the response to stimulation[86]. However, there are problems in defining what constitute resting conditions[86] and, owing to methodological difficulties, in deciding whether the changes with age represent increased production or diminished clearance of noradrenaline[115]. Wilkie *et al.*[116] found that plasma adrenaline, unlike noradrenaline, did not increase with age. There was, however, evidence for increased clearance of adrenaline, suggesting that secretion of the hormone must have risen similarly to maintain the plasma concentration.

Two studies have been done on the effects of elective surgery on plasma catecholamines in the elderly. Blichert-Toft *et al.*[101] found no difference in adrenaline or noradrenaline between old (aged 70–75) and young (aged 20–30) males, either basally or up to 6 hours after surgery. However, the operation, inguinal hernia repair, produced only a small and transient rise in the concentration of either catecholamine. After a more major operation, cholecystectomy, Håkanson *et al.*[106] found that the noradrenaline response was greater and much more prolonged (up to 48 hours instead of 2 hours) in patients aged 56–71 than in those aged up to 55, whereas the increase in adrenaline was small and transitory in both groups. No corresponding studies of accidental injury appear to have been published, but we have found that, within 3 hours of receiving severe accidental injuries (ISS $\geqslant$ 13), the plasma adrenaline and noradrenaline concentrations were raised similarly in patients aged 16–40 and in those aged over 65. Data unselected for age have been published[117]. The duration of the responses was not studied. Clearly, more work is needed before general statements can be made on the effects of ageing on the sympatho-adrenal response to trauma.

The sympatho-adrenal system is thought to be an influence, though not the only one, on the secretion of insulin and glucagon (discussed in the next section) and on the renin–angiotensin system after trauma. Plasma renin activity (PRA) decreases with age, probably owing to decreased distensibility of the renal juxtaglomerular apparatus[118]. In what appears to be the only relevant study of trauma, Blichert-Toft *et al.*[101] also found a lower basal PRA in elderly than in young patients, but in neither group did it respond to inguinal herniorrhaphy. Aldosterone, in contrast, rose transiently in both groups, with no difference between them. The results in younger patients are compatible with other studies, which show that aldosterone responds much more consistently to elective surgery than does PRA, and may often be due to ACTH instead of angiotensin II[83].

Metabolic response

In discussing the metabolic response to injury we shall continue to make the distinction between ebb and flow phases identified above for energy expenditure. Surprisingly little work has been done on the effects of ageing on this response. What little we know about the changes in fat metabolism all applies to the ebb phase, while our knowledge of the effects of injury on protein metabolism in the elderly is confined to the flow phase. The changes in carbohydrate metabolism, however, have been studied in both phases and we shall therefore start with a brief review of the extensive literature on the normal effects of ageing on the regulation of glucose homeostasis. An important consideration throughout this section is that body composition changes greatly with age, with a progressive rise in the proportion of fat at the expense of protein. This loss of lean body mass represents decreases in the size of most major tissues apart from the heart and lungs[51]. These changes may account for some of the apparent effects of ageing, and must be taken into consideration in extrapolating results from isolated tissues to the whole body.

Effect of ageing on carbohydrate metabolism

The work done up to 1979 has been comprehensively reviewed by Davidson[119]. Many studies have shown that there is a consistent but small increase in the fasting circulating glucose concentration with age, and a larger impairment of glucose tolerance. The insulin response to oral glucose tends to be greater but some reports have shown that old age decreases insulin secretion after intravenous glucose. Two studies used the hyperglycaemic clamp technique, in which glucose is infused at a variable rate so as to maintain a constant hyperglycaemia, but the conclusions disagreed; one showed a greatly decreased insulin response to the hyperglycaemia[120], whereas the other did not[121]. De Fronzo[121] did, however, find that insulin was less effective in stimulating whole-body glucose uptake in the elderly.

Since 1979, this insulin resistance has been put on a more quantitative basis by the development of the euglycaemic clamp, in which insulin is infused at a constant rate together with glucose at a rate that is continually varied so that the blood glucose concentration is kept at basal. Suppression of hepatic glucose production by this procedure is not substantially impaired in the elderly[121,122]. The dose-response curve (glucose utilization v. insulin concentration) was always shifted to the right in the elderly, implying insulin insensitivity, but there was disagreement over whether maximal responsiveness was also decreased[122–124]. Some decrease in responsiveness might be expected from the fall in lean body mass with age, but this was not the whole explanation[122]. The results of a number of studies suggest that the loss of sensitivity to insulin lies at the level of glucose transport across the cell membrane but that, unlike the loss of insulin sensitivity associated with obesity, it does not involve loss of insulin receptors[119,122,124–126]. However, there are problems in the interpretation of these studies. Those in man are of adipose tissue, which may not be typical of the insulin-dependent tissues as the relationship of its glucose uptake with insulin concentration, at least *in vitro*, is affected by age very differently from that in the whole body[126]. The metabolism of muscle, the major insulin-dependent tissue, has been studied in the rat, but the changes with age were largely confined to the first 16 weeks of life and may not have been relevant to the gradual effects of ageing in man[119,125].

Euglycaemic glucose clamps have also allowed the effects of ageing on whole-body insulin clearance to be measured. All the relevant studies have shown some decrease in insulin clearance in the elderly, but they disagree over whether this applies across the whole range of insulin concentrations or only at the lower infusion rates[122,127,128]. Other controlled studies done recently complement the results from euglycaemic clamps. Jackson *et al.*[129]

showed that, during oral glucose tolerance tests, forearm glucose uptake was lower in old than in younger men even if the latter were infused with glucose to give similar glucose and insulin concentrations; hepatic glucose uptake was unchanged but again insulin extraction decreased with ageing. From a 'minimal model' approach to interpreting intravenous glucose tolerance tests, Chen *et al.*[130] concluded that impairments of insulin secretion and action were important features of ageing whereas changes in insulin clearance and non-insulin-dependent glucose uptake were not.

Ageing and the ebb phase

The metabolic changes during the ebb phase can be seen as a response to the general activation of neuroendocrine systems. Identification of the hormones responsible for particular changes is difficult because many of them have similar effects. The most conspicuous feature is mobilization of body fuels[131]. Liver and probably muscle glycogen are broken down, resulting directly or indirectly in an increase in hepatic glucose output. The resulting hyperglycaemia fails to cause the expected increase in plasma insulin owing to α_2-adrenergic inhibition of insulin secretion, and is probably reinforced by insulin resistance[132]. The plasma glucose concentration rises exponentially with the ISS, although it is very variable at all values[107]. A similar relationship is seen for lactate[107], which is derived partly from glucose metabolism by hypoxic or glycolytic tissues and partly from any muscle glycogen breakdown that occurs. Triacylglycerol in adipose tissue is also broken down[131], but the plasma concentrations of the products of this lipolysis, glycerol and free fatty acids (FFA), do not increase consistently with ISS; in fact, plasma FFA is lower in patients with severe injuries than in those with moderate ones, perhaps because of impaired adipose tissue blood flow[107]. There is controversy over whether or not the concentrations of ketone bodies always follow those of FFA[131].

We and our colleagues have extended the observations of Stoner *et al.*[107] and have now examined the differences between age groups in the concentrations of various plasma constituents within the first hours of accidental injury, the severity of which has been assigned to one of three categories according to the ISS. There was a slightly but significantly greater hyperglycaemia in elderly (age >65) than in young (age 17–30) patients with minor injuries (ISS 1–6). Otherwise there were no differences in plasma glucose, insulin, lactate or alanine between these two age groups in any severity range. In contrast, the concentrations of all three lipid metabolites – glycerol, FFA and total ketone bodies (β-hydroxybutyrate plus acetoacetate) – tended to be higher in the elderly at all injury severities. The differences were greater for glycerol and total ketones, where the median values in the elderly were around twice those in the young, than they were for FFA. However, the values in all the groups were extremely variable and the differences were not always significant, especially for the severely injured (ISS ≥13) where the number of elderly patients was small.

There are two reports of the effects of ageing on the early metabolic responses to elective surgery, which usually causes smaller changes than accidental injury. Blichert-Toft *et al.*[101] found no significant difference in plasma glucose or insulin between elderly (age 70–75) and young (age 20–30) men undergoing inguinal hernia repair, although during the operation insulin tended to be lower in the elderly and postoperatively glucose tended to be higher. The latest samples were taken 6 hours postoperatively. Håkanson *et al.*[106] also found no difference in glucose or insulin concentrations between patients below and above 55 years of age during cholecystectomy or up to 4 days afterwards. They also measured alanine, lactate, glycerol, FFA and β-hydroxybutyrate. Of these only lactate showed any age-related differences; it tended to be higher in the elderly than in the younger patients, although significantly so only at 2 hours after skin incision when it was raised in both groups. However, there were differences between the sexes for glycerol, which was higher throughout (including preoperatively) in women than in men, and for FFA, which was also higher in women 2–4 days after surgery.

These studies agree in showing little effect of ageing on the changes in glucose or insulin during the ebb phase. This is perhaps surprising, as one might expect to see some influence of the age-related changes in carbohydrate metabolism outlined above. The reasons why such effects were not seen may have been different in the various studies; Håkanson *et al.*[106] found higher noradrenaline levels in the elderly after surgery whereas Blichert-Toft *et al.*[101] found no age-related differences in adrenaline or noradrenaline, and neither did we in our patients with severe accidental injuries; determinations of catecholamines were too few to make such comparisons in less severely injured patients. Given a similar sympatho-adrenal response, the results suggest that the effects of injury overrode the more subtle changes in carbohydrate metabolism that occur with normal ageing. For example, adrenergic inhibition was probably the dominant influence on insulin secretion, and might be little affected by age; similarly the age-related decrease in glucose transport might cause little further impairment of glucose utilization than that produced by injury, at least part of which is at a step beyond transport[133]. Ageing also had little effect on the plasma lactate concentration after injury. This suggests that the use of lactate to predict survival in various forms of shock[134] may not be valid at this stage after injury in the elderly, whose prognosis for a given ISS or type of operation is poorer than in younger patients. However, interpretation of lactate concentrations in the elderly is complicated by the decreased proportion of glycolytic Type II fibres in their skeletal muscle [135].

In contrast to carbohydrate metabolism, the effects of ageing on the changes in lipid metabolites were different in the two studies in which they were measured. Håkanson *et al.*[106] found similar responses to injury in young and old despite higher noradrenaline levels in the elderly, suggesting decreased sensitivity to noradrenaline. We found the opposite: concentrations of fat metabolites were higher in older patients despite a sympatho-adrenal response that appeared, at least in the severely injured, to be similar. Some of this apparent age difference could in fact be an effect of sex, since the great majority of our elderly patients were female whereas nearly all the young ones were male. However, the sex-related differences found by Håkanson *et al.*[106] are unlikely to account for all the discrepancies between the two studies. Further explanation is difficult as the literature on the effects of ageing on the products of lipolysis is incomplete and contradictory. Most studies have shown a tendency for the basal concentrations of FFA, glycerol and ketone bodies to increase with age[119,129,136,137]. Klein *et al.*[138], who studied FFA and glycerol kinetics isotopically, found that ageing had no significant effect either on the concentrations of FFA or glycerol or on their rates of production (unless expressed per unit mass of body fat). However, their results suggested that in those elderly subjects with high FFA concentrations (the values were very variable), these were due to decreased clearance rather than increased production. The number of β-adrenergic receptors in adipose tissue declines with age, in common with many other hormone receptors[139], and many studies *in vitro*, using adipose tissue mostly from animals, have shown a decrease in lipolysis in response to catecholamines and other stimuli[50,140]. However, corresponding changes do not yet appear to have been demonstrated in man *in vivo*. There is no difference between old and younger people in the increase in FFA caused by noradrenaline infusion[141] or starvation[138], nor does ageing affect the suppression of lipolysis by glucose administration[119].

Lipid mobilization has also been the subject of some of the very few studies of ageing using animal models of trauma. Hrůza and Jelínková[142] found that the increase in plasma FFA after Noble–Collip drum trauma was smaller in 1- or 2-year-old rats than in 7- to 10-week-old ('young') or 20-week-old ('adult') rats, despite their higher body fat content. Trauma also caused no increase in the FFA content of the periovarian or mesenteric fat depots in the older rats, in contrast to the adult ones. This was attributed to a lower response to catecholamines since a similar age difference in plasma FFA was seen after administration of adrenaline. Similar results were also seen with experimental turpentine abscess[143] and ageing reduced the rise in glucose and pyruvate but not lactate concentrations after this form of stress.

Ageing and the flow phase

Besides the increase in metabolic rate that gives it its name, the flow phase is characterized by an increase in net breakdown of protein in uninjured muscle, leading to an increase in nitrogen excretion greater than that caused by a similar period of reduced food intake[144] or immobility[145]. The cause of this response is not clear[132] but the carbon skeletons of the amino acids are presumably used to synthesize glucose, for which healing tissues have an obligatory requirement[46]. One would imagine that this need would be undiminished in old age.

There appears to be only one report of studies specifically on the effect of ageing on this protein catabolic response. Stableforth[146] found that in nearly all elderly women with fractures of the femoral neck the cumulative nitrogen balance over the first eight days was negative. All patients underwent surgery within 12 hours of injury, and the nitrogen balance was most negative in those requiring the most major operations. In addition, the nitrogen balance was positively correlated with the nitrogen intake, which varied considerably between patients, some of whom were given milk-based diet supplements. Comparison with the equivalent published relationships for younger women under-going major upper abdominal surgery showed that, although the slope was similar (around 5, indicating that intake of 1 g nitrogen and associated calories spared around 5 g body nitrogen), the elevation of the regression line was greater in the elderly patients, i.e. for a given nitrogen intake their nitrogen excretion was lower. This was attributed to a smaller surgical stress and to smaller labile protein stores resulting from a lower pre-traumatic protein intake. The author implied that age *per se* did not affect the response. As mentioned above, Carli and Itiaba[81] showed that heat conservation during major abdominal surgery reduced the subsequent increase in urinary nitrogen and 3-methylhistidine excretion, but they did not compare their elderly patients with younger ones.

The post-traumatic increase in nitrogen excretion represents the difference between the rates of protein breakdown and synthesis. Both rates increase with the degree of trauma but protein synthesis is very sensitive also to nutritional intake, leading to a complex set of relationships[147]. Makrides[148] has reviewed the large number of studies on the effects of ageing on protein synthesis and degradation in isolated tissues, mostly from animals. Nearly all show a decrease in protein turnover, an exception being the only study reported on human skeletal muscle. Golden and Waterlow[149] measured whole-body protein synthesis in normal elderly subjects by several methods and found rates that were probably lower than in younger subjects. Uauy *et al.*[52], who used the [^{15}N]glycine technique and included younger subjects in their study, confirmed this difference and showed by measuring 3-methylhistidine excretion that the decrease in protein breakdown (and by implication synthesis) was proportionately greater in skeletal muscle than elsewhere in the body. Whether it was greater than expected from the age-related loss of protein, i.e. whether it reflected the results with most *in vitro* preparations, is not clear. Clague *et al.*[147] consider that the decrease in protein turnover with age is due to a reduced nitrogen intake and predict that ageing, like other conditions associated with decreased protein turnover, will reduce the net nitrogen loss after trauma. The data of Stableforth[146] point in this direction, but studies using comparable degrees of trauma at different ages are needed.

The post-traumatic increase in net muscle protein breakdown is accompanied by peripheral insulin resistance, which may share a common stimulus[132]. In elderly patients with fractures of the femoral neck, the only group in which flow-phase changes in carbohydrate metabolism appear to have been studied, this insulin resistance was even more evident. The plasma glucose concentration was higher than in younger patients, even with injuries of greater ISS, for 2–3 weeks after trauma while plasma insulin was similar (and higher than in younger control subjects for reasons that are unclear)[109]. Clearly the age-related changes in carbohydrate metabolism may have contributed to these observations, but there is evidence that other factors were also involved. A role for immobility was suggested by the finding that inactive elderly control subjects had glucose and insulin levels tending to be even higher than those in the femoral fracture patients, whereas active ones had much lower levels[109]. Both insulin-resistant groups also had higher cortisol concentrations, suggesting that cortisol, which causes insulin resistance at physiological concentrations in man[150], could have mediated these effects of immobility. If so, the mechanism would have been different from that in young healthy subjects, in whom immobility causes peripheral insulin resistance but does not usually raise plasma cortisol[111]. Both increased cortisol concentrations[150] and greater immobility[145] would be expected to increase net muscle protein breakdown.

Another phenomenon of the flow phase is a set of characteristic changes in plasma proteins, of which many, the acute-phase reactants, increase in concentration while others, particularly albumin, decrease[151]. Little is known about the influence of age on these responses. In humans, the C-reactive protein response to clinically apparent infections appears well preserved[152,153]. We are not aware of any relevant studies in experimental animals. Gersovitz *et al.*[154] have shown that normal elderly and younger subjects have similar rates of albumin synthesis. This does not imply a similar fall in albumin concentration during the first few days after trauma as this fall is largely due to increased microvascular permeability rather than changes in synthesis or degradation[151]. However, the similar synthesis rate suggests that the subsequent recovery of albumin concentration will be unimpaired in the elderly.

Comprehensive studies of albumin metabolism in WAG/Rij rats during ageing[155] show a different picture from that in man. Although albumin concentration in the blood is not affected by ageing, there is a clear age-related increase in albumin elimination. This is matched by increased rates of albumin synthesis and albumin mRNA concentration in the liver, though the mRNA of the old animals appears to be biologically inferior.

The reticuloendothelial system

The reticuloendothelial system (RES) was originally described by Aschoff[156] as a system of mobile and fixed macrophages and specialized endothelial cells which together contribute to the natural resistance of a mammalian host to pathogenic microbes. Over the ensuing years, this description has had to be modified with regard to both cellular composition and function.

In his original description, Aschoff classified the cellular constituents of the RES as follows:

1. Reticular cells of lymphoid organs.
2. Endothelial cells of hepatic lobules (Kupffer cells).
3. Connective tissue histiocytes.
4. Splenocytes.
5. Monocytes.

Nowadays, Kupffer cells are known to be of the macrophage lineage and display phagocytic activity, as do all other macrophages. Notwithstanding, true endothelial cells (particularly those in the liver) contribute to the capacity of the RES to clear the circulation of a variety of materials by non-phagocytic uptake processes.

Functions of the RES

As mentioned above, the most prominent and best studied function of the RES is the capacity to clear the circulation of many materials, including inert colloids, tissue debris, bacteria and bacterial endotoxins[157]. Most of this clearance function is concentrated in the Kupffer cells and endothelial cells of the hepatic sinusoid[158].

Macrophage clearance of gelatinized test particles is influenced by plasma fibronectin[159,160]. Fibronectin binds to fibrin, actin, collagen and heparin[161] and has been suggested to play a role in promoting RES clearance of fibrin, collagenous debris and cytoskeletal debris following injury. It is known that the concentration of fibronectin is diminished by extensive trauma, starvation, disseminated intravascular coagulation and experimental RES blockade[161]. It is known to increase in cirrhosis, obstructive jaundice and advanced age[162,163].

Cells of the RES also participate in immune responses and can present antigens[164–166]. These cells are also secretory cells and release enzymes such as collagenase and lysosomal enzymes, free radicals, interleukin-1, prostaglandins and leukotrienes, procoagulant factors, interferons, colony-stimulating factors and tumoricidal factors[167].

Secretory products of the RES may be involved in some of the metabolic changes observed after injury and may even contribute to tissue damage. One substance that has attracted considerable interest is 'macrophage insulin-like activity'[168]. There is clear evidence that it contributes to the hypoglycaemia seen in endotoxin shock. Other substances may modulate hepatocyte protein synthesis. Keller and co-workers[169–171] have shown that soluble factors secreted by Kupffer cells can do so and that they are similar but not identical to interleukin-1. Leukotrienes are produced by many RES cells and can cause liver damage[172]. Leukotrienes C4 and D4 can induce endothelial cells to secrete platelet-activating factor[173] and this can cause ischaemic injury, including bowel necrosis[174].

Many factors are capable of modulating RES activity but no comprehensive, integrated picture of how the RES is regulated *in vivo* can yet be given. Glucocorticoids, several other hormones, vasoactive amines and peptides as well as poorly characterized splenic factors can all modify RES activity[157]. Furthermore, a variety of exogenous factors can be used experimentally to enhance or suppress RES activity[162].

Assessment of RES activity

Techniques to assess RES activity are mostly oriented towards its clearance function. Biozzi[175] was the first to introduce a reliable test and this is still used in a modified form. In brief, a large dose of colloid (calculated to exceed the maximum rate of clearance) is injected intravenously and blood samples are collected at intervals. The concentrations are plotted semi-logarithmically against time and the resulting disappearance curve usually follows first-order kinetics. The half-life time or the phagocytic index can then be calculated, though more complex calculations can be made to take into account variations in dose, liver size, spleen size and blood flow.

The requirements for an appropriate test colloid were summarized by Benacerraf[176] as follows. The colloid should be:

1. Stable.
2. Homogeneous in size.
3. Non-toxic.
4. Taken up only by RES cells.
5. Unaltered by contact with blood.

In clinical practice, especially after trauma or in the presence of sepsis, large doses of test colloid cannot be given because of the theoretical risk that they may depress RES activity (RES blockade). Preliminary studies using low doses of technetium tin colloid in rabbits suggest that this substance might be useful for assessing RES activity in a clinical setting[177]. The only other techniques commonly used in man are the injection of ^{125}I- or

[131]I-labelled microaggregates of denatured human serum albumin, the injection of ^{131}I-labelled RE test lipid emulsion and the measurement of plasma fibronectin.

Injury and RES function

Very soon after ischaemic injury, trauma or circulatory shock of any kind, RES function as assessed by colloid clearance is depressed and damage to endothelial cells is apparent[157,178]. Regardless of the nature or aetiology of the injury or shock, the degree of RES depression is directly related to its severity[157,178]. The reduction in colloid clearance can be detected within 30 minutes of injury. In subjects destined not to survive, this RES depression persists until death whereas survivors display a progressive recovery of clearance capacity which frequently rises above basal between days 1 and 4 after injury with a return to normal at 4–5 days[178–180]. Plasma fibronectin concentration appears faithfully to reflect these changes[181].

RES *blockade* with colloidal carbon or large doses of choline chloride has the effect of increasing fatality among experimental animals subjected to several shock models[179,182]. Furthermore, the histamine H_2-receptor antagonist burinamide resulted in RES depression with similar consequences[183]. RES stimulation with low-dose choline chloride, denatured albumin, triolein, zymosan, glucan and low doses of endotoxins has a protective effect in several shock models[157,178], though, for some unknown reason, not all of these substances protect in all models. Pharmacological doses of glucocorticoids and oestrogens, vasopressin and its synthetic analogues, α-adrenergic blockers, opiate antagonists, H_1 histamine receptor antagonists, quinones, and non-steroidal anti-inflammatory agents also protect in animal shock models[178] though all these substances have actions other than RES stimulation through which their effects could be mediated.

Although attention is often focused on the actively phagocytic cells of the RES, changes in endothelial cells may be critical in the pathogenesis of some of the ischaemic damage that may be seen after injury. Indeed, it has already been stated that endothelial cell damage and dysfunction are very early events in the shock syndrome, and at this time the peripheral vasculature overcompensates and produces severe ischaemia in the gut, liver and kidneys. This led Altura[178] to propose that early endothelial cell injury/dysfunction influences the response of vascular smooth muscle to vasoactive substances. Convincing evidence was provided by *in vivo* quantitative TV image-intensification microscopic techniques and showed that normally vasodilative mediators could produce vasoconstriction under these circumstances. The precise mechanism of these effects is not yet known.

Ageing and the RES

A number of investigators have used colloid-clearance techniques to investigate the influence of age on RES function in man. Studies using colloidal gold[184,185], aggregated albumin[186] and technetium sulphur colloid[184] have all demonstrated an age-related prolongation of half-life time. According to Brouwer and Knook[187], this represents a 15% decline in clearance between the ages of 30 and 80. Brouwer and Knook[187] also re-calculated some of the data of Wagner and co-workers[186] and suggested that the age-related decline in RES activity could be as well explained by changes in blood-flow characteristics as by intrinsic changes in the cells themselves.

The literature on the effects of ageing on RES function in experimental animals has been extensively reviewed by Brouwer and Knook[187]. The data are sparse as well as contradictory and some of the contradictions can be explained by flaws in methodology. On balance, it is safe to conclude that there is a definite but small decline in the clearance capacity of the RES during ageing and this is supported by work published by Brouwer and Knook[188] themselves. They showed that the maximal rate of endocytosis of ^{125}I-labelled colloidal albumin by cultured Kupffer cells was decreased in cells obtained from 30- to 36-month-old rats when compared with cells from animals aged 3 months. Intermediate age groups gave intermediate results. Values for K_m, which gives an indication of the affinity of the cells for the ligand, were not affected by age.

Aoki and co-workers[189] reported that administration of zymosan to aged mice did not result in as great an enhancement of RES activity as was observed in younger animals. This confirms the observations of Old et al.[190] but contradicts those of Di Carlo et al.[191]. These studies on the effects of age on the ability to modulate RES activity are perhaps more relevant to a discussion on injury responses than observations made in a basal state.

Ageing and the response to endotoxins

Endotoxins are lipopolysaccharide components of the cell walls of Gram-negative bacteria. They are biologically extremely active substances, with a wide spectrum of target organs and tissues, and are widely used in experimental shock research. They are rapidly taken up by mononuclear phagocytes and the RES appears to provide the only route for their elimination[192]. Furthermore, products of RES cells seem to be critical in the pathogenesis of endotoxin toxicity[193,194]. One fascinating feature of endotoxin toxicity is the wide variation in sensitivity observed in different species. For example, guinea-pig > hamster > mouse > rat. This sensitivity profile correlates with the rate of phagocytosis of latex particles by Kupffer cells and with the numbers of Kupffer cells in the hepatic lobule[195]. Guinea-pigs have the fastest rate of phagocytosis and the highest Kupffer cell density.

All the observations just described suggest that endotoxins would provide a useful model for the testing of injury responses in an experimental setting, not only because of the important role of the RES but also because a whole variety of host defences are triggered and the possibly deleterious effects of ageing in individual systems might be expected to be exposed.

Habicht[59] reported that aged C57 BL/6 mice showed a considerably greater mortality rate after endotoxin administration than their younger counterparts and that this increased mortality was associated with disordered thermoregulation. These observations were confirmed by Hoffman-Goetz and Keir[57]. We have observed the same phenomenon in ageing rats from two strains (BN/BiRij and WAG/Rij) and both sexes[162]. Indeed, there was hardly any overlap of mortality curves of 3- and 6-month-old animals with those of 24- and 36-month-old animals. Intermediate responses were seen in 18-month-old animals. This increased fatality was associated with profound hypothermia and hypoglycaemia together with hypercoagulability of the blood[196]. The plasma half-life of endotoxin was also significantly prolonged in the older animals, but not markedly so[197,198], suggesting that phagocytic activity is not critical to the lethal effects of endotoxins. These older animals also showed much more severe histopathological changes, particularly in the kidneys, liver, adrenals and lungs[162,196,199]. The pulmonary damage is particularly interesting in the light of the discussion above on the role of endothelial cells since the lung injury occurred within 15–30 minutes and affected predominantly pulmonary endothelial cells. It was concluded that the pulmonary endothelial cells of aged rats are more susceptible to endotoxin-induced injury and that platelets play a role in the enhancement of the initial damage to the endothelium.

The responses of aged rodents to endotoxin administration

appear to provide a good example of the concept that we proposed in the Introduction above: responses in the intact organism may be more fundamental in ageing research than changes at the molecular level. These observations are also exciting since there appears to be a possibility for therapeutic intervention by pharmacological manipulation of RES activity. Perhaps the most important question for further research is which RES activities to attempt to modulate. Phagocytic activity is but little affected by ageing and cannot explain the age-related increase in sensitivity to the lethal effects of endotoxins. We feel that further investigations into the secretory products of the RES are likely to be more fruitful.

Conclusion

In the Introduction we postulated that minor deteriorations with age in individual physiological or biochemical systems would have a more than additive effect when the body was exposed to the major disruption of injury. One might expect this to be most pronounced in the early ebb phase and to be reflected in a large increase in fatality during the first 24 hours after injury. It is not clear from published data whether this is so, but a recent study suggested that appreciable numbers of old people even with very severe injuries survive this period[200]. Certainly, the available evidence shows that the elderly do not fail to mount an adequate neuroendocrine response to their injuries; the systems studied – mainly the sympatho-adrenal system and hypothalamus–pituitary–adrenal axis – show changes at least as great as those in younger patients. While some of the effects of these neuroendocrine changes are probably diminished, this is not true of all of them; the ability of the elderly injured patient to mobilize his or her glycogen and fat stores appears to be at least equal to that of the young one. Much more information is needed in all these areas, but our tentative conclusion is that the ageing body copes surprisingly well with the acute insult of injury.

The same cannot be said of the chronic effects of injury. Morbidity and fatality are increased, and deaths continue for a long period after injuries that would not normally be considered severe[2–4,26,27]. While part of this must be due to pre-existing disease and malnutrition, it is likely that age-related differences in injury responses contribute. In the elderly patient with a fracture of the neck of the femur, there is evidence for peripheral insulin resistance which may be associated with a prolonged rise in plasma cortisol and with immobility[109]. However, the nature of these interrelationships is not understood, nor is it clear whether they represent cause or effect or neither. The insulin resistance suggests a greater disturbance in skeletal muscle metabolism than in younger patients, and one might expect to see a larger net breakdown of protein. However, the very limited data available suggest that the protein catabolic response is decreased in line with muscle mass and previous nutritional intake[146]. Clearly, far more work is needed in this area. There are obvious implications for therapy, particularly in terms of nutrition.

Several studies suggest the potential for improvement in the nutrition of the elderly trauma patient. Bastow and co-workers[201] showed that elderly women with evidence of antecedent malnutrition had a higher fatality rate after fracture of the femoral neck than their well-nourished counterparts. Intervention in the form of supplementary nasogastric feeding in these malnourished patients, who also ate less after their injury, reduced fatality from 22% to 8%, although this was not statistically significant[202]. In the malnourished patients who survived, supplementary nutrition reduced the time they needed to remain in hospital. Allison[72] suggested that such therapy would only be of benefit in patients with severe nutritional depletion, but Stableforth[146] has shown supplementary feeding to cause considerable improvements in nitrogen balance in elderly hip-fracture patients unselected for nutritional status.

Deficiencies in nutrition also contribute to the impaired ability of the elderly to regulate their body temperature[72,201]. This impairment is of particular interest in view of the changes that characterize both phases of the response to injury, as well as playing a possible role in its pathogenesis[72,201]. The possible relevance to therapy is illustrated by the work of Carli and Itiaba[81], who showed that minimizing heat loss during major surgery decreased the subsequent nitrogen loss in elderly patients. However, the changes in thermoregulation are another example of what is true of all aspects of the response to injury: far too little is known about the effects of ageing. The provision of this knowledge should be a major challenge to those who recognize the need for improving the care of the elderly trauma patient on a scientific basis.

Acknowledgements

We should like to thank Dr K. N. Frayn and Professor H. B. Stoner for their help in obtaining unpublished data mentioned in this review.

References

1. COMFORT, A. *Gerontologia*, **14**, 224 (1968)
2. SEYMOUR, G. *Medical Assessment of the Elderly Surgical Patient*, Croom Helm, London (1986)
3. TUBBS, N. *Injury*, **7**, 233 (1976)
4. BULL, J. P. *Accid. Anal. Prev.*, **7**, 249 (1975)
5. HORST, H. M., OBEID, F. N., SORENSEN, V. J. *et al. Crit. Care Med.*, **14**, 681 (1986)
6. EVANS, J. G., PRUDHAM, D. and WANDLESS, I. *Publ. Health (London)*, **93**, 235 (1979)
7. REES, J. L. *Comm. Med.*, **4**, 100 (1982)
8. KNOWELDEN, J., BUHR, A. J. and DUNBAR, O. *Br. J. Prev. Soc. Med.*, **18**, 130 (1964)
9. BAKER, M. R. *Publ. Health (London)*, **94**, 368 (1980)
10. LEWIS, A. F. *Br. Med. J.*, **283**, 1217 (1981)
11. EVANS, J. G. *Lancet*, **1**, 925 (1985)
12. BALDWIN, J. A. *Br. Med. J.*, **284**, 271 (1982)
13. HEDLUND, R., AHLBOM, A. and LINDGREN, U. *Acta Orthop. Scand.*, **57**, 30 (1985)
14. BOYCE, W. J. and VESSEY, M. P. *Lancet*, **1**, 150 (1985)
15. MELTON, L. J., WAHNER, H. W., RICHELSON, L. S. *et al. Am. J. Epidemiol.*, **124**, 254 (1986)
16. GRIBBIN, B., PICKERING, J. G., SLEIGHT, P. *et al. Circ. Res.*, **29**, 424 (1971)
17. WILLIAMS, B. O., CAIRD, F. I. and LENNOX, I. M. *Age Ageing*, **14**, 193 (1985)
18. ROWE, J. W., MINAKER, K. L., SPARROW, D. *et al. J. Clin. Endocrinol. Metabol.*, **54**, 661 (1982)
19. HRŮZA, Z. and ZWEIFACH, B. W. *J. Gerontol.*, **22**, 469 (1967)
20. DASTUR, D. K., LANE, M. H., HANSEN, D. B. *et al.* In *Human Aging, a Biological and Behavioral Study* (ed. J. E. Birren, R. N. Butler, S. W. Greenhouse *et al.*), PHS Publication No. 986, Washington, DC, US Government Printing Office, p. 59 (1963)
21. DUARA, R., LONDON, E. D. and RAPOPORT, S. I. In *Handbook of the Biology of Aging*, 2nd edn (ed. C. E. Finch and E. L. Schneider), Van Nostrand Reinhold, New York, p. 595 (1985)
22. HAINING, J. L., TURNER, M. D. and PANTALL, R. M. *Am. J. Physiol.*, **218**, 1020 (1970)
23. BAKER, S. P., O'NEILL, B. and HADDON, W. *J. Trauma*, **14**, 187 (1974)
24. CHAMPION, H. R., SACCO, W. J., CARNAZZO, A. J. *et al. Crit. Care Med.*, **9**, 672 (1981)
25. KNAUS, W. A., DRAPER, E. A., WAGNER, D. P. *et al. Crit. Care Med.*, **13**, 818 (1985)
26. HOLMBERG, S., CONRADI, P., KALÉN, R. *et al. Acta Orthop. Scand.*, **57**, 8 (1986)
27. JENSEN, J. S. and TÖNDEVOLD, E. *Acta Orthop. Scand.*, **50**, 161 (1979)
28. WILMORE, D. W. *The Metabolic Management of the Critically Ill*, Plenum, New York (1977)
29. MITCHELL, H. H. *Comparative Nutrition of Man and Domestic Animals*, vol. 1, Academic, New York (1962)
30. CUTHBERTSON, D. P. *Lancet*, **1**, 433 (1942)
31. STONER, H. B. *J. Appl. Physiol.*, **33**, 665 (1972)
32. STONER, H. B. In *Homeostasis in Injury and Shock. Advances in Physiological Sciences*, vol. 26 (ed. Zs. Bíró, A. G. B. Kovách, J. J. Spitzer *et al.*), Akadémiai Kiadó, Budapest, p. 25 (1981)

33. STONER, H. B. In *The Scientific Basis for the Care of the Critically Ill* (ed. R. A. Little and K. N. Frayn), Manchester University Press, Manchester, p. 215 (1986)
34. STONER, H. B. *Br. J. Exp. Pathol.*, **50**, 125 (1969)
35. LITTLE, R. A., STONER, H. B. and FRAYN, K. N. *Clin. Sci.*, **61**, 789 (1981)
36. LITTLE, R. A. *Br. Med. Bull.*, **41**, 226 (1985)
37. LITTLE, R. A. and STONER, H. B. *Br. J. Surg.*, **68**, 221 (1981)
38. LITTLE, R. A., MARSHALL, H. W., REYNOLDS, M. I. *et al. Pflügers Arch.*, **384**, 261 (1980)
39. LITTLE, R. A., STONER, H. B., RANDALL, P. *et al. Q. J. Exp. Physiol.*, **71**, 295 (1986)
40. FRAYN, K. N., LITTLE, R. A., STONER, H. B. *et al. Injury*, **16**, 73 (1984)
41. DAVIES, J. W. L. *Physiological Responses to Burning Injury*, Academic, New York (1982)
42. CLIFTON, G. L., ROBERTSON, C. S. and CHOI, S. C. *J. Neurosurg.*, **64**, 895 (1986)
43. LITTLE, R. A. In *Update in Intensive Care and Emergency Medicine (Update 3)* (ed. J. L. Vincent), Springer-Verlag, Berlin, p. 16 (1987)
44. WILMORE, D. W., LONG, J. M., MASON, A. D. *et al. Ann. Surg.*, **180**, 653 (1974)
45. AULICK, L. H., HANDER, E. H., WILMORE, D. W. *et al. J. Trauma*, **19**, 559 (1979)
46. WILMORE, D. W. In *The Scientific Basis for the Care of the Critically Ill* (ed. R. A. Little and K. N. Frayn), Manchester University Press, Manchester, p. 45 (1986)
47. STONER, H. B. *Circ. Shock*, **19**, 75 (1986)
48. MATSON, J. R. and HITCHCOCK, F. A. *Am. J. Physiol.*, **110**, 329 (1934)
49. DURNIN, J. V. G. A. *Br. J. Nutr.*, **13**, 68 (1959)
50. GREGERMAN, R. I. and BIERMAN, E. L. In *Textbook of Endocrinology*, 6th edn (ed. R. H. Williams), Saunders, Philadelphia, p. 1192 (1981)
51. RUDMAN, D. *J. Am. Geriat. Soc.*, **33**, 800 (1985)
52. UAUY, R., WINTERER, J. C., BILMAZES, C. *et al. J. Gerontol.*, **33**, 663 (1978)
53. SHOCK, N. W. In *Handbook of the Biology of Aging* (ed. C. E. Finch and L. Hayflick), Van Nostrand Reinhold, New York, p. 639 (1977)
54. KIANG-ULRICH, M. and HORVATH S. M. *Exp. Gerontol.*, **20**, 107 (1985)
55. HOFFMAN-GOETZ, L. and KEIR, R. *J. Gerontol.*, **39**, 547 (1984)
56. TOCCO-BRADLEY, R., SINGER, R., KLUGER, M. J. *et al. Gerontology*, **31**, 349 (1985)
57. HOFFMAN-GOETZ, L. and KEIR, R. *J. Gerontol.*, **40**, 15 (1985)
58. TALAN, M. I. and INGRAM, D. K. *Mech. Age Develop.*, **33**, 247 (1986)
59. HABICHT, G. S. *Mech. Age Develop.*, **16**, 97 (1981)
60. HORVATH, S. M., RADCLIFFE, C. E., HUTT, B. K. *et al. J. Appl. Physiol.*, **8**, 145 (1955)
61. COLLINS, K. J., EXTON-SMITH, A. N. and DORÉ, C. *Br. Med. J.*, **282**, 175 (1981)
62. MACMILLAN, A. L., CORBETT, J. L., JOHNSON, R. H. *et al. Lancet*, **2**, 165 (1967)
63. COLLINS, K. J., DORÉ, C., EXTON-SMITH, A. N. *et al. Br. Med. J.*, **1**, 353 (1977)
64. KRAG, C. L. and KOUNTZ, W. B. *J. Gerontol.*, **5**, 227 (1950)
65. LEAN, M. E. J. and JAMES, W. P. T. In *Brown Adipose Tissue* (ed. P. Trayhurn and D. G. Nicholls), Edward Arnold, London, p. 299 (1986)
66. BRUCK, K. In *Brown Adipose Tissue* (ed. O. Lindberg), Elsevier, New York, p. 117 (1970)
67. MARCHINGTON, D., ROTHWELL, N. J., STOCK, M. J. *et al. Am. J. Physiol.*, **250**, E362 (1986)
68. LE FEUVRE, R. A., ROTHWELL, N. J. and STOCK, M. J. *Neuropharmacology*, **26**, 1217 (1987)
69. FINCH, C. E., FOSTER, J. R. and MIRSKY, A. E. *J. Gen. Physiol.*, **54**, 690 (1969)
70. LETO, S., KOKKONEN, G. C. and BARROWS, C. H. *J. Gerontol.*, **31**, 144 (1976)
71. FELLOWS, I. W., MACDONALD, I. A., BENNETT, T. *et al. Clin. Sci.*, **69**, 525 (1985)

72. ALLISON, S. P. In *The Scientific Basis for the Care of the Critically Ill* (ed. R. A. Little and K. N. Frayn), Manchester University Press, Manchester, p. 169 (1986)
73. COLLINS, K. J. In *The Nature and Treatment of Hypothermia* (ed. R. S. Pozos and L. E. Wittmers), Croom Helm, London, p. 257 (1983)
74. ROTHBAUM, D. A., SHAW, D. J., ANGELL, C. S. *et al. J. Gerontol.*, **29**, 488 (1974)
75. WEISFELDT, M. L., LOEVEN, W. A. and SHOCK, N. W. *Am. J. Physiol.*, **220**, 1921 (1971)
76. MUIESAN, G., SORBINI, C. A. and GRASSI, V. *Bull. Physio-Pathol. Resp.*, **7**, 973 (1971)
77. KLOCKE, R. A. In *Handbook of the Biology of Aging* (ed. C. E. Finch and L. Hayflick), Van Nostrand Reinhold, New York, p. 432 (1977)
78. NIINIMAA, V. and SHEPHARD, R. J. *J. Gerontol.*, **33**, 362 (1978)
79. SHOCK, N. W. In *Nutrition in Old Age (X Symposium of the Swedish Nutrition Foundation)* (ed. L. A. Carlson), Almqvist & Wiksells, Stockholm, p. 12 (1972)
80. RENCK, H. *Acta Anaesthesiol. Scand.,* Suppl. 34 (1969)
81. CARLI, F. and ITIABA, K. *Br. J. Anaesth.*, **58**, 502 (1986)
82. GANN, D. S. and AMARAL, J. F. In *The Management of Trauma*, 4th edn (ed. G. D. Zuidema, R. B. Rutherford and W. F. Ballinger), Saunders, Philadelphia, p. 37 (1985)
83. BARTON, R. N. *Baillière's Clin. Endocrinol. Metabol.*, **1**, 355 (1987)
84. DAVIS, P. J. *Clin. Endocrinol. Metabol.*, **8**, 603 (1979)
85. GREGERMAN, R. I. *Exp. Gerontol.*, **21**, 345 (1986)
86. ROWE, J. W. and TROEN, B. R. *Endocrine Rev.*, **1**, 167 (1980)
87. ROGERS, J. and BLOOM, F. E. In *Handbook of the Biology of Aging,* 2nd edn (ed. C. E. Finch and F. L. Schneider), Van Nostrand Reinhold, New York, p. 645 (1985)
88. WEST, C. D., BROWN, H., SIMONS, E. L. *et al. J. Clin. Endocrinol. Metabol.*, **21**, 1197 (1961)
89. SERIO, M., PIOLANTI, P., CAPPELLI, G. *et al. Exp. Gerontol.*, **4**, 95 (1969)
90. FRIEDMAN, M., GREEN, M. F. and SHARLAND, D. E. *J. Gerontol.*, **24**, 292 (1969)
91. BLICHERT-TOFT, M., BLICHERT-TOFT, B. and KAALUND JENSEN, H. *Acta Chir. Scand.*, **136**, 665 (1970)
92. MONCLOA, F., GÓMEZ, R. and PRETELL, E. *Steroids*, **1**, 437 (1963)
93. BLICHERT-TOFT, M. *Acta Endocrinol.* (Suppl. 195), **78**, 1 (1975)
94. TOURIGNY-RIVARD, M-F., RASKIND, M. and RIVARD, D. *Biol. Psychiat.*, **16**, 1177 (1981)
95. PAVLOV, E. P., HARMAN, S. M., CHROUSOS, G. P. *et al. J. Clin. Endocrinol. Metabol.*, **62**, 767 (1986)
96. BLICHERT-TOFT, M. and HUMMER, L. *Gerontology*, **23**, 236 (1977)
97. ROMANOFF, L. P., MORRIS, C. W., WELCH, P. *et al. J. Clin. Endocrinol. Metabol.*, **21**, 1413 (1961)
98. SAPOLSKY, R. M., KREY, L. C. and McEWEN, B. S. *Endocrine Rev.*, **7**, 284 (1986)
99. PEKKARINEN, A., VIIKARI, S. and TURUNEN, M. *Ann. Med. Exp. Biol. Fenn.* (Suppl. 7), **35**, 1 (1957)
100. NILSSON, E., ARNER, B. and HEDNER, P. *Acta Chir. Scand.*, **126**, 281 (1963)
101. BLICHERT-TOFT, M., CHRISTENSEN, V., ENGQUIST, A. *et al. Ann. Surg.*, **190**, 761 (1979)
102. BLICHERT-TOFT, M. and HUMMER, L. *J. Gerontol.*, **31**, 539 (1976)
103. QUERIDO, A. and VAN SETERS, A. P. In *The Human Adrenal Cortex: its Function throughout Life* (Ciba Foundation Study Group No. 27) (ed. G. E. W. Wolstenholme and R. Porter), Churchill, London, p. 119 (1967)

104. BOWEN, D. J. and RICHARDSON, D. J. *Br. J. Anaesth.*, **46**, 873 (1974)
105. OYAMA, T., TANIGUCHI, K., TAKAZAWA, T. *et al. Can. Anaesth. Soc. J.*, **27**, 556 (1980)
106. HÅKANSON, E., RUTBERG, H., JORFELDT, L. *et al. Clin. Physiol.*, **4**, 461 (1984)
107. STONER, H. B., FRAYN, K. N., BARTON, R. N. *et al. Clin. Sci.*, **56**, 563 (1979)
108. BARTON, R. N., STONER, H. B. and WATSON, S. M. *J. Trauma*, **27**, 384 (1987)
109. FRAYN, K. N., STONER, H. B., BARTON, R. N. *et al. Age Ageing*, **12**, 70 (1983)
110. BARTON, R. N. and STONER, H. B. *Circ. Shock*, **21**, 292 (abstract 1) (1987)
111. VERNIKOS, J. In *Inactivity: Physiological Effects* (ed. H. Sandler and J. Vernikos), Academic, Orlando, Fla, p. 99 (1986)
112. EVERITT, A. V. and BURGESS, J. A. In *Hypothalamus Pituitary and Aging*, Thomas, Springfield, Ill., p 464 (1976)
113. LE QUESNE, L. P., COCHRANE, J. P. S. and FIELDMAN, N. R. *Br. Med. Bull.*, **41**, 212 (1985)
114. YOUNG, J. B., ROSA, R. M. and LANDSBERG, L. *Am. J. Physiol.*, **247**, E35 (1984)
115. CHRISTENSEN, N. J. *Eur. J. Clin. Invest.*, **12**, 91 (1982)
116. WILKIE, F. L., HALTER, J. B., PRINZ, P. N. *et al. J. Gerontol.*, **40**, 133 (1985)
117. FRAYN, K. N., LITTLE, R. A., MAYCOCK, P. F. *et al. Circ. Shock*, **16**, 229 (1985)
118. FRANKLIN, S. S. *Med. Clin. North Am.*, **67**, 395 (1983)
119. DAVIDSON, M. B. *Metabolism*, **28**, 688 (1979)
120. ANDRES, R., POZEFSKY, T., SWERDLOFF, R. S. *et al. Adv. Metabol. Disorders*, Suppl. 1, 349 (1970)
121. DE FRONZO, R. A. *Diabetes*, **28**, 1095 (1979)
122. FINK, R. I., KOLTERMAN, O. G., GRIFFIN, J. *et al. J. Clin. Invest.*, **71**, 1523 (1983)
123. ROWE, J. W., MINAKER, K. L., PALLOTTA, J. A. *et al. J. Clin. Invest.*, **71**, 1581 (1983)
124. PAGANO, G., CASSADER, M., CAVALLO-PERIN, P. *et al. Metabolism*, **33**, 976 (1984)
125. GOODMAN, M. N., DLUZ, S. M., McELANEY, M. A. *et al. Am. J. Physiol.*, **244**, E93 (1983)
126. FINK, R. I., KOLTERMAN, O. G., KAO, M. *et al. J. Clin. Endocrinol. Metabol.*, **58**, 721 (1984)
127. MINAKER, K. L., ROWE, J. W., TONINO, R. *et al. Diabetes*, **31**, 851 (1982)
128. REAVEN, G. M., GREENFIELD, M. S., MONDON, C. E. *et al. Diabetes*, **31**, 670 (1982)
129. JACKSON, R. A., BLIX, P. M., MATTHEWS, J. A. *et al. J. Clin. Endocrinol. Metabol.*, **55**, 840 (1982)
130. CHEN, M., BERGMAN, R. N., PACINI, G. *et al. J. Clin. Endocrinol. Metabol.*, **60**, 13 (1985)
131. BARTON, R. N. *Br. Med. Bull.*, **41**, 218 (1985)
132. FRAYN, K. N. *Clin. Endocrinol.*, **24**, 577 (1986)
133. HEATH, D. F. In *The Scientific Basis for the Care of the Critically Ill* (ed. R. A. Little and K. N. Frayn), Manchester University Press, Manchester, p. 75 (1986)
134. VITEK, V. and COWLEY, R. A. *Ann. Surg.*, **173**, 308 (1971)
135. HALJAMÄE, H., STEFÁNSSON, T. and WICKSTRÖM, I. *Acta Anaesthesiol. Scand.*, **26**, 393 (1982)
136. ALBERTI, K. G. M. M., DORNHORST, A. and ROWE, A. S. *Biochem. Soc. Trans.*, **3**, 132 (1975)
137. FOSTER, K. J., ALBERTI, K. G. M. M., HINKS, L. *et al. Clin. Chem.*, **24**, 1568 (1978)
138. KLEIN, S., YOUNG, V. R., BLACKBURN, G. L. *et al. J. Clin. Invest.*, **78**, 928 (1986)
139. ROTH, G. S. *Fed. Proc.*, **38**, 1910 (1979)
140. MASORO, E. J., BERTRAND, H., LIEPA, G. *et al. Fed. Proc.*, **38**, 1956 (1979)
141. EISDORFER, C., POWELL, A. H., SILVERMAN, G. *et al. J. Gerontol.*, **20**, 511 (1965)
142. HRŮZA, Z. and JELÍNKOVÁ, M. *Gerontologia*, **8**, 36 (1963)
143. HRŮZA, Z., JELÍNKOVÁ, M. and HLAVÁČKOVÁ, V. *Exp. Gerontol.*, **1**, 127 (1965)

144. CUTHBERTSON, D. and TILSTONE, W. J. *Adv. Clin. Chem.*, **12**, 1 (1969)
145. CUTHBERTSON, D. P. In *Mammalian Protein Metabolism*, vol. 2 (ed. H. N. Munro and J. B. Allison), Academic, New York, p. 373 (1964)
146. STABLEFORTH, P. G. *Br. J. Surg.*, **73**, 651 (1986)
147. CLAGUE, M. B., KEIR, M. J., WRIGHT, P. D. *et al. Clin. Sci.*, **65**, 165 (1983)
148. MAKRIDES, S. C. *Biol. Rev.*, **58**, 343 (1983)
149. GOLDEN, M. H. N. and WATERLOW, J. C. *Clin. Sci. Mol. Med.*, **53**, 277 (1977)
150. GELFAND, R. A., MATTHEWS, D. E., BIER, D. M. *et al. J. Clin. Invest.*, **74**, 2238 (1984)
151. FLECK, A., COLLEY, C. M. and MYERS, M. A. *Br. Med. Bull.*, **41**, 265 (1985)
152. KENNY, R. A., HODKINSON, H. M., COX, M. L. *et al. Age Ageing*, **13**, 89 (1984)
153. COX, M. L., RUDD, A. G., GALLIMORE, R. *et al. Age Ageing*, **15**, 257 (1986)
154. GERSOVITZ, M., MUNRO, H. N., UDALL, J. *et al. Metabolism*, **29**, 1075 (1980)
155. HORBACH, G. J. M. J. Albumin metabolism and aging. *PhD Thesis*, State University of Limburg (1986)
156. ASCHOFF, L. *Ergebn. Inn. Med. Kinderheilkd.*, **26**, 1 (1925)
157. ALTURA, B. M. In *Advances in Microcirculation*, vol. 9, (ed. B. M. Altura), Karger, Basle, p. 252 (1980)
158. BROUWER, A., BARELDS, R. J., DE LEEUW, A. M. *et al.* In *Pharmacological, Morphological and Physiological Aspects of Liver Aging* (ed. C. F. A. Van Bezooijen), Eurage, Rijswijk, p. 181 (1983)
159. SABA, T. M., BLUMENSTOCK, F. A., WEBER, P. *et al. Ann. NY Acad. Sci.*, **312**, 43 (1978)
160. BLUMENSTOCK, F. A., SABA, T. M., ROCCARIO, E. *et al. J. Reticuloendoth. Soc.*, **30**, 61 (1981)
161. YAMADA, K. M. and OLDEN, K. *Nature*, **275**, 179 (1978)
162. HORAN, M. A. Endotoxin as a naturally occurring immunomodulator. *PhD Thesis*, State University of Utrecht (1986)
163. STATHAKIS, N. E., FOUNTAS, A. and TSIANOS, E. *J. Clin. Pathol.*, **34**, 504 (1981)
164. UNANUE, E. R. *Adv. Immunol.*, **15**, 95 (1972)
165. ROSENTHAL, A. S. *N. Engl. J. Med.*, **303**, 1153 (1980)
166. ROGOFF, T. M. and LIPSKY, P. E. *Gastroenterology*, **80**, 854 (1981)
167. PAGE, R. C., DAVIES, P. and ALLISON, A. C. *Int. Rev. Cytol.*, **52**, 119 (1978)
168. FILKINS, J. P., JANUSEK, L. W. and YELICH, M. R. In *Bacterial Endotoxins and Host Response* (ed. M. K. Agarwal), Elsevier/North Holland, Amsterdam, p. 361 (1980)
169. KELLER, G. A., WEST, M. A., CERRA, F. B. *et al. Ann. Surg.*, **201**, 87 (1985)
170. KELLER, G. A., WEST, M. A., WILKES, L. A. *et al. Ann. Surg.*, **201**, 429 (1985)
171. KELLER, G. A., WEST, M. A., HARTY, J. T. *et al. Ann. Surg.*, **201**, 436 (1985)
172. HAGMANN, W., DENZLINGER, C. and KEPPLER, D. *FEBS Lett.*, **180**, 309 (1985)
173. McINTYRE, T. M., ZIMMERMAN, G. A. and PRESCOTT, S. M. *Proc. Natl Acad. Sci. USA*, **83**, 2204 (1986)
174. HSUEH, W., GONZALEZ-CRUSSI, F. and ARROYAVE, J. L. *Am. J. Pathol.*, **122**, 231 (1986)
175. BIOZZI, G., BENACERRAF, B. and HALPERN, B. N. *Br. J. Exp. Pathol.*, **34**, 441 (1953)
176. BENACERRAF, B. In *The Liver*, vol. II (ed. E. Rouiller), Academic, New York, p. 37 (1964)
177. CHADWICK, S. J. D., ALDRIDGE, M. and DUDLEY, H. A. F. *Br. J. Exp. Pathol.*, **66**, 483 (1985)
178. ALTURA, B. M. In *The Scientific Basis for the Care of the Critically Ill* (ed. R. A. Little and K. N. Frayn), Manchester University Press, Manchester, p. 259 (1986)

179. ALTURA, B. M. and HERSHEY, S. G. *J. Reticuloendoth. Soc.*, **10**, 361 (1971)
180. ALTURA, B. M. and HERSHEY, S. G. *Proc. Soc. Exp. Biol. Med.*, **139**, 935 (1972)
181. RICHARDS, P. S. and SABA, T. M. *Hepatology*, **5**, 32 (1985)
182. FILKINS, J. P. *J. Reticuloendoth. Soc.*, **22**, 461 (1977)
183. ALTURA, B. M. and HALEVY, S. *Proc. Natl Acad. Sci. USA*, **75**, 2941 (1978)
184. MUNDSCHENK, H., HROMEC, A. and FISCHER, J. *J. Nucl. Med.*, **12**, 711 (1971)
185. ANTONINI, F. M., CAPPELLI, G., CITI, S. *et al. J. Gerontol.*, **12**, 741 (1964)
186. WAGNER, H. N., MIGITA, T. and SOLOMON, N. *J. Gerontol.*, **21**, 57 (1966)
187. BROUWER, A. and KNOOK, D. L. *Mech. Age Devel.*, **21**, 205 (1983)
188. BROUWER, A. and KNOOK, D. L. *J. Reticuloendoth. Soc.*, **32**, 259 (1982)
189. AOKI, T., TELLER, M. N. and ROBITAILLE, M-L. *J. Natl Cancer Inst.*, **34**, 255 (1965)
190. OLD, L. J., CLARKE, D. A., BENACERRAF, B. *et al. Ann. NY Acad. Sci.*, **88**, 264 (1960)
191. DI CARLO, F. J., HAYNES, L. J. and PHILLIPS, G. E. *Proc. Soc. Exp. Biol. Med.*, **112**, 651 (1963)
192. MATHISON, J. C. and ULEVITCH, R. J. *J. Immunol.*, **123**, 2133 (1979)
193. MATHISON, J. C. and ULEVITCH, R. J. *Surv. Synth. Pathol. Res.*, **1**, 34 (1983)
194. FILKINS, J. P. *Fed. Proc.*, **44**, 300 (1985)
195. McCUSKEY, R. S., McCUSKEY, P. A., URBASCHEK, R. *et al. Infect. Immunol.*, **45**, 278 (1984)
196. BROUWER, A., HORAN, M. A., BARELDS, R. J. *et al. Age* (in press)
197. HORAN, M. A., BROUWER, A., BARELDS, R. J. *et al.* In *Cells of the Hepatic Sinusoid*, vol. 1 (ed. A. Kirn, D. L. Knook and E. Wisse), Kupffer Cell Foundation, Rijswijk, p. 303 (1986)
198. BROUWER, A., HORAN, M. A., BARELDS, R. J. *et al. Arch. Gerontol. Geriat.*, **5**, 317 (1986)
199. HENDRIKS, H. F. J., HORAN, M. A., DURHAM, S. K. *et al. Mech. Age Devel.*, **41**, 241 (1988)
200. FIFE, D. *Injury*, **18**, 315 (1987)
201. BASTOW, M. D., RAWLINGS, J. and ALLISON, S. P. *Lancet*, **1**, 143 (1983)
202. BASTOW, M. D., RAWLINGS, J. and ALLISON, S. P. *Br. Med. J.*, **287**, 1589 (1983)

Chapter 10

Joint replacement in the elderly

I. G. Kelly

Introduction

The past 20 years have seen the development and proliferation of surgical techniques for the replacement of arthritic joints. The late Sir John Charnley was the most notable pioneer, and he established the requirements for the successful replacement of the hip joint. He was particularly concerned with the behaviour of these replacements in patients of different ages and stated that 'over the age of 70 . . . this is the age group where total hip replacement is one of the greatest boons to mankind'[1]. The same sentiment can now be expressed for replacement of other joints.

But what constitutes an elderly patient? Chronological age is certainly not, *per se*, a contraindication to surgery or anaesthesia. The physiological age, reflected by the manifestations of the ageing process, is the most relevant in this respect. It may, however, be difficult to ascertain – 'age is not dependent on years, but on temperament and health' (Tyron Edwards). When I asked colleagues what they thought of as an elderly patient, the most useful answer I received in relation to joint replacement was 'a patient whose life expectancy is not sufficient to have to consider revision of the arthroplasty'. Using this definition 'elderly' could have different implications for patients undergoing replacement of different joints and is related to the actuarial concept of life expectancy. Rather than discuss a particular age group in what follows I will consider the physiological changes that take place during the ageing of the musculoskeletal system and relate them to the performance of joint replacement.

Indications for surgery

There are many causes for an arthritic joint, e.g. osteoarthritis, rheumatoid arthritis and previous fracture, but the general principles of joint replacement are the same in every case.

The aim of joint replacement in any patient is the restoration of function. In the 'elderly' this frequently equates with the maintenance of an independent lifestyle. The fundamental indication for surgery in this group is therefore the loss of function sufficient to interfere with an independent existence.

Many factors affect function. Pain is probably the most important and indeed the decision to carry out joint replacement at most sites depends largely upon its severity. However, a note of caution must be sounded here. Pain in relation to joints, especially in the lower limbs, may be a result of other conditions which may be present in the older patient. For example, peripheral vascular disease may produce claudication in the buttock or thigh and Paget's disease, a common condition, may also produce pain distinct from that which may result from any co-existent degree of degenerative change in the adjacent joint. Function may also be affected by co-existent cardiovascular disease, limiting walking distance, and by disease in other joints, muscles or the central nervous system. The radiograph, generally thought of as the orthopaedic surgeon's *sine qua non*, is of limited value in these elderly patients since it has little part to play in deciding the indications for surgery and merely serves to guide the surgeon in his choice of procedure.

The indications for surgery must also include consideration of the patient's medical status. Multi-system disease is common with advancing years and may not always be obvious. A typical example is the patient with an arthritic hip and cardiovascular disease who cannot exercise sufficiently to load the myocardium to a stage that will produce symptoms. A thorough preoperative medical examination is therefore important and this must also include an investigation of the presence of occult infection, especially in the urinary tract. Such an infection may produce transient bacteraemia which can result in infection of the joint replacement.

A related problem is postoperative retention of urine in men. The incidence of prostatic hypertrophy is naturally very high in this group and the presence of the symptoms of prostatism are often overlooked, by both patient and physician. Anaesthetic drugs, analgesics, the pain of surgery and the postoperative recumbency can all contribute to retention of urine which may become chronic. The need for catheterization and perhaps even urological surgery all pose a great risk to the prosthesis from the point of view of infection. The presence of significant symptoms of prostatism should alert the surgeon to the possibility of this postoperative problem and a simple screening test has been described. If the patient can urinate into a bottle when lying supine then few postoperative problems are to be anticipated[2].

The effects of ageing on the musculoskeletal system

Ageing produces a loss of the physiological reserve function in any system. From the musculoskeletal point of view the major problems are osteoporosis and loss of muscle bulk.

Osteoporosis appears to be an inevitable part of ageing with a decrease in metabolic rate of both osteoblasts and osteoclasts occurring after the age of 40 years. Trabecular bone is lost early and when the cortex is affected endosteal loss takes place, resulting in a large medullary cavity in the long bones[3].

This change in quality affects the mechanical properties of bone. In particular, it becomes less elastic and therefore more brittle. Its resistance to stress declines and fractures are more likely to occur.

There is a loss in the number and size of muscle fibres[4]. In part this is a consequence of disuse atrophy but the effect is also seen in those who persist in rigorous physical activity. It is more marked in the lower limb than in the upper limb and is most pronounced in the proximal part of the limbs. There are also central effects which affect muscular and postural control. The latter appears to be a multifactorial problem, as much related to deficient afferent impulses – visual and proprioceptive – as to the central effects. With age the skeleton therefore becomes both more brittle and less well protected by its muscles and their control systems.

Joint replacement

Most joint replacements involve the use of a metallic component articulating with either bone – a 'hemi-arthroplasty' – or a polyethylene component – a total joint replacement. Components are fixed into the medullary cavity of the bone using polymethylmethacrylate bone cement, which is not a glue but acts as a grout. The major technical problem of joint replacement is to achieve and maintain effective fixation.

Fixation is a function of the efficacy of the methylmethacrylate–bone bond and the load to which this bond is subjected. As previously mentioned, osteoporosis has a particular effect on the endosteal bone, reducing its volume and increasing the volume of the medullary canal. Such capacious medullary cavities may not provide a secure fix for standard prosthetic stems and can make the alignment of the stems within them more difficult, thereby affecting the reconstruction of the joint. These factors prejudicial to fixation may be partly compensated for by the reduced muscle bulk and reduced activity of this group of patients which will result in lower loads being exerted upon the joint replacement.

Complications

The problems encountered after joint replacement are related to the joint which is being replaced, but there are a few complications common to all.

The incidence of infection following arthroplasty has been reduced to the order of 1% or less by the use of preoperative skin preparation, prophylactic antibiotics and clean air operating enclosures. The incidence of infection appears to be no higher in elderly patients.

Deep venous thrombosis (DVT) is a well-recognized complication, particularly of hip and knee joint arthroplasty, and an incidence of 54% in patients undergoing hip joint replacement has been reported[5]. There is some evidence that the risk of postoperative DVT increases with age[6] and preventive measures should always be considered in the elderly patient.

Methylmethacrylate has been associated with cardiovascular problems intraoperatively. Transient hypotension is not infrequently recorded[7] and complete circulatory collapse with cardiac arrest and death has been reported. The elderly patient with reduced cardiovascular reserve is obviously more at risk from this effect, which may be minimized by adequate intraoperative fluid replacement and oxygenation.

Rehabilitation

Inserting the arthroplasty is only a small part of the process of returning the patient to a functional state and an independent existence. The joint operated upon has a significant bearing upon the ease of rehabilitation. Typically, after total hip replacement the patient will be out of bed on the second or third day and walking with the assistance of walking aids and a physiotherapist by the fourth day. With a knee joint replacement, however, this may take considerably longer. Cooperation with the rehabilitation process is essential to obtain the best results irrespective of the age of the patient. Elderly patients, however, may be deaf, mildly demented or dysphasic. These factors must be recognized and time has to be spent before operation in ensuring that the patient understands what will be required after the surgery has been performed. It is important not to attempt to return the patient to the functional status of, for example, a young fit man. This is clearly unnecessary and impossible, and time spent in attempting to achieve it will be wasted, probably resented and will be positively harmful to morale. In most instances, as long as the patient can exist independently it matters little if activities such as dressing take as long as an hour.

The functional needs of every patient are different and the evaluation of the requirements of each individual necessitates an understanding of the patient's social background, lifestyle and environment. These features dictate that rehabilitation is carried out under the auspices of a team. The combined services of the medical social worker, the occupational therapist – in hospital and in the home – and the physiotherapist, in liaison with the general practitioner, hospital medical and nursing staff provide the support for effective rehabilitation.

Problems associated with individual joints

Specific problems are associated with particular joint replacements.

Hip joint

This is the most commonly replaced joint in the elderly with the best established form of implant and the most information regarding its efficacy. The problems of fixation as a result of osteoporosis have already been alluded to, but osteoporosis can also have an undesirable effect at a later stage and it is possible to sustain fractures below the prosthesis, often as a result of minor violence. This can be a particularly difficult situation to manage and may require further surgery.

Dislocation of the hip joint is a well-recognized complication, occurring in about 5% of patients. It is typically managed by the reduction of the hip joint and bed-rest for several weeks in traction. This is clearly undesirable in the elderly patient and a method has evolved which has minimized the period of recumbency. After a few days spent in bed it is possible to apply a splint to the thigh linked by a hinge to a belt worn round the waist. This device limits the ability of the hip to adduct and flex and therefore protects the joint from those movements most likely to produce dislocation. Within this brace the patient is free to walk and to be at home.

Knee joint

Replacement of the knee joint is not as well established as that of the hip joint but useful results can be achieved. One aspect that has been emphasized here is the undesirable effect of the use of the tourniquet. This can produce a degree of hypertension which in its turn may result in myocardial overload, especially when used in conjunction with narcotic nitrous oxide anaesthesia[8]. Post-operatively rehabilitation is very much more difficult than for the hip joint and a 3 week stay in hospital may well be required before the patient can cope at home even with the appropriate social support. Continued outpatient physiotherapy then presents the problem of travelling from home to hospital several times a week.

Shoulder and elbow

It is now possible to replace the upper limb joints, and although this is usually carried out in patients with rheumatoid arthritis many are elderly. Rehabilitation of the shoulder even in a young patient is a prolonged affair but need be no more difficult for elderly patients as long as they are able to cooperate with the rehabilitation regime, which requires that much of the exercising be done by the patient at home. The elbow joint presents fewer problems since there is usually a rapid return to full motion postoperatively.

Conclusion

The majority of patients undergoing joint replacement in this country are elderly. The indications differ little from those in the young, although in that group alternative procedures might well be considered in view of the finite lifetime of a joint replacement. There is only a slightly increased risk of complications and very few medical problems now contraindicate anaesthesia. Although rehabilitation may be slow, it is usually satisfactory, particularly when adequate information has been provided to the patient beforehand. The key to success is the relief of pain, which is associated with the restoration of a useful although usually limited range of movement. This allows the return of function and independence. Joint replacements do indeed seem to be 'one of the greatest boons to mankind'.

References

1. CHARNLEY, J. *Low Friction Arthroplasty of the Hip. Theory and Practice,* Springer-Verlag, Berlin (1979)
2. WATERHOUSE, N., BEAUMONT, A. R., MURRAY, K. *et al. J. Bone Joint Surg.,* **69B**, 64 (1987)
3. JOWSEY, J. *Metabolic Diseases of Bone,* Saunders, Philadelphia (1977)
4. TOGHI, H., SCHIMIZO, T., INOVE, K. and KAMEYAMA, M. *Clin. Neurol. (Tokyo),* **15**, 798 (1975)
5. LOUDEN, J. R., THORBURN, J., GRAHAM, J. *et al. Br. Med. J.,* **1**, 1550 (1978)
6. MORRELL, M. T., TRUELOVE, S. C. and BARR, A. *Br. Med. J.,* **2**, 830 (1963)
7. CHARNLEY, J. *Acrylic Cement in Orthopaedic Surgery,* Williams and Wilkins, Baltimore, Maryland (1970)
8. KAUFMAN, R. D. and WALTS, L. F. *Br. J. Anaesth.,* **54**, 334 (1982)

Chapter 11

Medical fitness for joint replacement

J. B. McDonald

Joint replacement has been one of medicine's most recent and outstanding successes. Historically there were many attempts at joint replacement before the recent development of durable alloys and bone cements, together with improved anaesthetic and surgical techniques, produced the current levels of success. Hip arthroplasty is now one of the more common elective surgical procedures and is performed predominantly for people aged 65 and over. The major indications for joint replacement are incapacitating pain and greatly restricted mobility. It is in the relief of these symptoms that joint replacement is so successful: pain is abolished in 90% of patients undergoing hip arthroplasty and mobility is significantly increased in 80%[1]. This improvement in function may be an underestimate, as the patient may be limited by pain in other joints or by unrelated pathology, for example cardiovascular or pulmonary disease.

The main diseases leading to hip arthroplasty – osteoarthritis and rheumatoid arthritis – are not in themselves life-threatening, whereas joint replacement surgery carries risks. Hip arthroplasty has a fatality of 1% to 5% and a morbidity rate of 5% to 10%[1]. The morbidity and fatality rates for knee joint replacement are slightly higher. However, medical treatment also is not without risk. About one-quarter of 'yellow card' reports of adverse drug reactions concern non-steroidal anti-inflammatory drugs[2]. These drugs are a cause of gastrointestinal bleeding[3] and possibly of upper gastrointestinal perforation[4]. They can also precipitate heart failure and have been implicated in renal failure. Clearly, the risks of medical management as well as the potential benefits of surgery must be weighed against the possible morbidity and fatality of surgical intervention.

Many aspects of medical assessment of elderly patients for surgery have been reviewed by Seymour[5,6]. Surgical risk may be reduced by improving surgical and anaesthetic techniques, by better postoperative care, and by improving the medical fitness of the patient. The physician involved in assessing medical fitness is not the arbiter of which patient should proceed to surgery; that decision rests with the surgeon. Nor should advice on anaesthetic techniques be offered to anaesthetic colleagues. The role of the physician is to evaluate the risk factors present, to correct those amenable to treatment and to identify those factors likely to cause complications perioperatively.

Age-associated changes occur in many of the organ systems that affect operative outcome, and lack of functional reserve explains why 'fit' older patients are at greater risk of operative complications than 'fit' younger patients[7]. On average, compared with younger subjects cardiac output in the elderly is reduced at rest and responds less well to stress[8]. The older patient is therefore less able to respond adaptively to changes in intravascular volume so that fairly small amounts of blood loss may cause a disproportionate degree of hypotension and a fairly small intravenous fluid overload may precipitate heart failure.

Age-associated changes in pulmonary function lead to a fall in arterial oxygen saturation and vital capacity[9], which can result postoperatively in restlessness from unsuspected hypoxia. Increase in colonization of the upper airways with Gram-negative bacilli may play a part in the genesis of postoperative chest infections[10]. In patients who are achlorhydric, or who are rendered so by therapy with H_2-blockers such as cimetidine or ranitidine, colonization of the upper airways and subsequent pneumonia may result from gastric regurgitation[11].

Bacteriuria increases in prevalence with age[12] and may predispose to pyelonephritis and bacteraemia. Urinary retention is a well-recognized postoperative complication in elderly men and may also affect elderly women, particularly if constipation is not recognized and treated. Age-associated decline in renal function may predispose to electrolyte imbalance and dehydration, particularly if diuretic therapy is used, and insensitivity of the thirst mechanism in elderly patients is a compounding factor[13].

The prevalence of autonomic dysfunction[14] and cognitive impairment[15] increase with age and can significantly affect postoperative rehabilitation. Both should be looked for before elective surgery so that problems can be avoided or anticipated.

Cardiovascular disease

Cardiovascular disease is one of the major predictors of outcome and those patients without overt cardiovascular risk factors have a low incidence of cardiovascular complications postoperatively[7]. Cole[16] identified left ventricular dysfunction and hypertension as poor prognostic indicators. This was confirmed by Del Guercio and Cohn[17], who studied 148 elderly patients using cardiac catheterization to detect cardiorespiratory pathology. They found that 25% of patients studied had abnormalities that made them unsuitable for general anaesthetic. All the patients in this category who proceeded to surgery against medical advice died. Goldman[7] identified a series of cardiac signs and symptoms which carried with them an increased risk of serious postoperative complications. The clinical signs most closely related to poor outcome were an elevated jugular venous pressure, a third heart sound and clinical and radiological signs of left heart failure. Elective surgery should not be undertaken until heart failure has been brought under control.

Recent myocardial infarction has been shown to be associated with an increased incidence of postoperative complications. Patients operated on within 3 months of a myocardial infarction have a reinfarction rate of around 30%, although by 6 months this risk has fallen to 4% to 5% and remains at that level[18,19]. However, a recent study[20] has not confirmed these observations and suggests that it is the extent of myocardial damage which is the important indicator rather than myocardial infarction itself.

Cardiac arrhythmias in patients with underlying heart disease also carry an increased risk of perioperative and postoperative complications[21,22]. Atrial fibrillation should be controlled and patients with heart disease and more than five ventricular beats per minute or runs of ventricular extrasystoles should be assessed for possible antiarrhythmic therapy.

There is widespread agreement that hypertension should be controlled before operation. The literature provides conflicting evidence regarding the pressure at which intervention becomes appropriate. Goldman and Caldera[23] suggest that there is no increased risk if blood pressure is below 180/110 mmHg but not all the patients in the series reported were elderly. Other investigators have suggested that postoperative risk begins to increase with the pressure above 180/100[16].

Several attempts have been made to combine the various cardiovascular findings into a composite predictive index for preoperative surgical assessment. Little work has been done that is specific to elderly patients, and none of the indices is yet very satisfactory[6].

The incidence of postoperative stroke in surgical patients aged 65 and over is variously estimated as between 4 and 33 per thousand[6]. This may be compared with an incidence in the general population aged 65 and over of 11 to 25 per thousand per year[24]. Little has been written about the risks of surgery after stroke and there is no clear evidence that a history of previous stroke increases the risk perioperatively[6]. Although one might suspect that the hormonal changes, the increase in platelet stickiness and the possible increase in blood viscosity that occur perioperatively might compound pre-existing risk factors for stroke, this does not appear to have been rigorously documented. It seems prudent to postpone elective surgery for 6 months after a stroke, to ensure that the patient's clinical condition is stable and that any risk from a possible underlying cardiac cause, particularly 'silent' infarction, is minimized. Neurological disability is not in itself a bar to joint replacement. If the condition is stable and there is no other contraindication, the patient should be allowed to proceed to surgery but the need for intensive postoperative remobilization anticipated.

Other factors

Anaemia must be assessed for both its functional significance and its possible aetiology. A haemoglobin of 10 g/dl is generally accepted as a safe minimum level for patients with a normal blood volume and good cardiovascular and respiratory function[25]. A haematocrit of 50% or higher should alert the physician to the possibility of underlying disease and is a warning that special care must be taken to ensure that the patient does not become dehydrated with an associated increase in blood viscosity. The evidence of increased postoperative risk associated with polycythaemia is most firmly based on a study of patients with polycythaemia rubra vera[26] and the value of venesection for patients with secondary polycythaemia has not been established.

Chest disease will have an important influence on postoperative management and anaesthetic technique. A preoperative assessment of the degree or reversibility of airway obstruction may be of value in perioperative management. The introduction of spinal anaesthesia has allowed surgery to a group of patients who in the past might have been denied its potential benefits.

Diabetes mellitus signifies an increased risk of cardiovascular complications and if not properly controlled may predispose to poor wound healing and to infection and postoperative hyperosmolar syndrome. Safe control requires a blood glucose running at around 12 mmol/l[27]. Measurement of blood rather than urine glucose is necessary as an elevated renal threshold is common in the elderly. It is wise to control blood glucose with intravenous insulin by infusion in the perioperative period in diabetics. The presence of infection preoperatively must be avoided. The skin should be examined to ensure there is not intertrigo and the urine examined to exclude infection.

Poor nutrition is seldom a problem in elderly people who do not have diseases such as malignancy or dementia that may exclude them from consideration for joint replacement. Although the major problems related to obesity occur with upper abdominal and thoracic surgery, an orthopaedic surgeon will often require a grossly obese patient to lose weight before embarking on joint replacement.

Who should do the assessment?

For most patients the initial screening can be simple. A full history and clinical examination including blood pressure lying and standing and a formalized assessment of mental function are required. Investigations can normally be limited to a full blood count, blood glucose, urea and electrolytes, mid-stream assessment of urine, chest X-ray and ECG. These investigations are readily available to most general practitioners and if the screening is conscientiously carried out only those patients with abnormal findings need to be referred for the opinion of a consultant physician. The screening should be done within about 8 weeks of planned surgery, although up to 3 months is acceptable. Other approaches have been described[28] and combined medical-surgical assessment clinics could prove very effective in those settings where firm 'diary' bookings for operations can be made by orthopaedic surgeons at the time of first referral of patients[29]. It is clearly highly desirable that factors affecting the risk of complications to surgery should be identified as part of a preliminary assessment and not when the patient is admitted for surgery.

References

1. LIANG, H. L., CULLEN, K. E. and POSS, R. *Ann. Intern. Med.*, **97**, 735 (1982)
2. LANGMAN, M. J. S. *Adv. Drug React. Bull.*, **120**, 448 (1968)
3. SOMERVILLE, K., FAULKNER, G. and LANGMAN, M. *Lancet*, **1**, 462 (1986)
4. WALT, R., KATSCHINSKI, B., LOGAN, R. *et al. Lancet*, **1**, 489 (1986)
5. SEYMOUR, D. G. In *Advanced Geriatric Medicine 3* (ed. F. I. Caird and J. G. Evans), Pitman, London, p. 163 (1983)
6. SEYMOUR, G. *Medical Assessment of the Elderly Surgical Patient*, Croom Helm, London (1986)
7. GOLDMAN, L. *Ann. Intern. Med.*, **98**, 504 (1983)
8. LAKATTA, E. G., *J. Chron. Dis.*, **36**, 15 (1983)
9. SORBINI, C. A., GRASSI, V., SOLINAS, E. and MUIESAN, G. *Respiration*, **25**, 3 (1968)

10. VALENTI, W. M., TRUDELL, R. G. and BENTLEY, D. M. *N. Engl. J. Med.*, **298**, 1108 (1978)
11. DRIKS, M., CRAVEN, D. E., CELLI, B. R. *et al. N. Engl. J. Med.*, **317**, 1376 (1987)
12. DONTAS, A. S. In *Urology in the Elderly* (ed. J. C. Brocklehurst), Churchill Livingstone, Edinburgh, p. 162 (1984)
13. PHILLIPS, P. A., ROLLS, B. J., LEDINGHAM, J. G. G. *et al. N. Engl. J. Med.*, **311**, 753 (1984)
14. COLLINS, K. J., EXTON-SMITH, A. N., JAMES, M. H. and OLIVER, D. J. *Age Ageing*, **9**, 17 (1980)
15. ROYAL COLLEGE OF PHYSICIANS WORKING PARTY. *J. R. Coll. Phys. Lond.*, **15**, 3 (1981)
16. COLE, W. H. *Ann. Surg.*, **168**, 310 (1968)
17. DEL GUERCIO, L. R. M. and COHN, J. D. *JAMA*, **243**, 1350 (1980)
18. STEEN, P. A., TINKER, J. H. and TARHAN, S. *JAMA*, **239**, 2566 (1978)
19. TARHAN, S., MOFFIT, E. A., TAYLOR, W. F. and GIULIANI, E. R. *JAMA*, **220**, 1451 (1972)
20. FOSTER, A. *Ann. Thorac. Surg.*, **41**, 42 (1986)
21. GOLDMAN, L., CALDERA, D. L., NUSSBAUM, S. R. *et al. N. Engl. J. Med.*, **297**, 845 (1977)
22. SEYMOUR, D. G., PRINGLE, R. and MACLENNAN, W. J. *Age Ageing*, **12**, 97 (1983)
23. GOLDMAN, L. and CALDERA, D. L. *Anesthesiology*, **50**, 285 (1979)
24. EVANS, J. G. *J. Epidemiol. Commun. Hlth*, **41**, 275 (1987)
25. RAWSTRON, R. E. *Anaesth. Intensive Care*, **4**, 175 (1976)
26. WASSERMAN, L. R. and GILBERT, H. S. *Ann. NY Acad. Sci.*, **115**, 122 (1964)
27. BAGDADE, J. D., ROOT, R. K. and BULGER, R. J. *Diabetes*, **23**, 9 (1974)
28. DEVAS, M. In *Geriatric Orthopaedics* (ed. M. Devas), Academic Press, London, p. 1 (1977)

Chapter 12

Calcium antagonists and angiotensin converting enzyme inhibitors in the elderly

M. Hardman

It might be argued that one does not have to understand the workings of the internal combustion engine to be able to drive a car. By analogy one does not have to understand the pharmacology of drugs to be able to prescribe them. However, a basic understanding of the mechanisms of action of drugs undoubtedly allows the prescriber to use drugs more appropriately and more safely.

Calcium antagonists

Calcium passes through the cell membrane via several pharmacologically distinct channels[1]. Two calcium channels are insensitive to calcium antagonists, a calcium–sodium counter-transport channel and a passive diffusion channel. Two channels are sensitive to calcium antagonists, a potential (voltage)-operated channel sensitive to the extracellular potassium concentration and a receptor-modulated channel sensitive to noradrenaline (NA). Angiotensin II (AII) and 5-hydroxytryptamine (5-HT) facilitate NA release whilst dopamine is inhibitory. An increase in intracellular calcium induces the sequence: calcium–calmodulin complex formation, activation of myosin light-chain kinase, phosphorylation of myosin and muscle contraction. Relaxation depends on the dephosphorylation of myosin and/or the inactivation of myosin light-chain kinase which is brought about by beta-adrenoceptor activation.

Calcium antagonists are chemically heterogeneous (Figure 12.1), and include dihydropyridines (nifedipine and nitrendipine), phenylalkylamines (verapamil) and benzothiazepines (diltiazem). It is generally accepted that the dihydropyridines bind to a specific receptor and that the non-dihydropyridines allosterically regulate this binding site, although the exact pharmacology is far from clear. The differences between tissues in the number of binding sites and their affinity for calcium antagonists partly explains the specificity of action of the different drugs. For example,

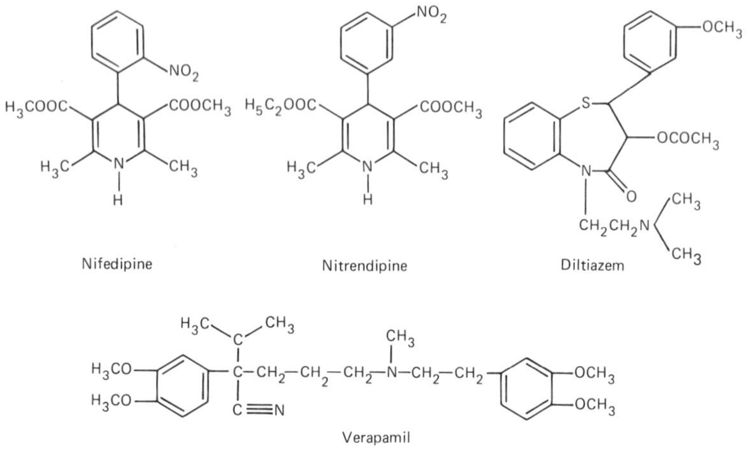

Nifedipine

Nitrendipine

Diltiazem

Verapamil

Figure 12.1 Structure of some calcium antagonists, demonstrating the heterogeneity of this group of drugs

verapamil has a much greater effect on the atrioventricular node in the heart than nifedipine, which exerts its major effects on peripheral blood vessels and is therefore an antihypertensive rather than an antiarrhythmic. There are differential sites of action within the vasculature; diltiazem is more selective for the coronary arteries, whereas nimodipine dilates venous vessels. The future of calcium antagonists will no doubt revolve around increasingly specific drugs for individual vascular beds.

Since the function of all cells is modulated by calcium fluxes it is not surprising that calcium antagonists have been tried in many clinical conditions. Table 12.1 summarizes some of the clinical indications currently being explored. The three most widely accepted uses for calcium antagonists are angina, hypertension and cardiac arrhythmias.

Angina

Calcium antagonists have been shown to be efficacious in elderly patients and with few adverse cardiovascular or other side-effects[2]. There are two aspects of angina, spasm of the coronary arteries (with or without associated atheromatous disease), giving unstable angina, and chronic stable angina associated with fixed arterial stenoses. Patients with unstable angina exhibit diurnal variation in symptoms. Spasm of the coronary arteries typically occurs in the middle of the night and this is thought to be due to

Table 12.1 Calcium antagonists: indications under clinical investigation

Cardiovascular

  Ischaemic heart disease
    angina pectoris
    myocardial infarction
        acute treatment
        prevention
  Cardiac arrhythmias
  Systemic arterial hypertension
  Hypertrophic cardiomyopathy
  Congestive cardiac failure
  Pulmonary hypertension
  Raynaud's syndrome
  Disturbances in cerebral perfusion
  Atherogenesis

Non-cardiovascular

  Bronchial asthma
  Smooth muscle spasm
    intestine
    gallbladder
    ureter
    oesophagus
    bladder detrusor
  Premature labour
  Dysmennorhoea
  Ergotism
  Increasing anti-tumour activity of vinca alkaloids

changes in extracellular pH. Experimentally it can be shown that increasing the extracellular pH increases the tension in vascular smooth muscle and that this increase is calcium-dependent[3]. In a clinical study of a patient with typical unstable angina[3], hyperventilation, causing a rise in arterial pH, was associated with coronary spasm and myocardial ischaemia manifested as raised ST segments on the electrocardiogram. These changes were prevented by prior treatment with diltiazem.

Calcium antagonists are the drugs of choice in unstable angina since they comprise the only group that consistently reduces rather than exacerbates coronary artery spasm (Table 12.2). In chronic stable angina, there is little or no scope for dilating the stenosed coronary arteries, but calcium antagonists may produce benefit by relaxing coronary vascular tone in the myocardial penetrating arteries and capillary bed, and by reducing end-diastolic pressure through systemic peripheral vasodilatation. These two effects

Table 12.2 Effects of various drugs on the attacks induced by treadmill exercise in patients with variant angina[2]

ST-segment elevation	Propanolol (%)	Diltiazem (%)	Nifedipine (%)	Phentolamine (%)
Suppressed completely	0	77	87	42
Improved by more than 0.1 mV	17	23	13	39
Improved by less than 0.1 mV	41	0	0	11
Aggravated by more than 0.1 mV	42	0	0	8

increase the blood flow to the compromised subendothelial myocardium[4].

Hypertension

A small increase in intracellular calcium is amplified by a further release of calcium from the smooth endoplasmic reticulum (the vast majority of intracellular calcium is bound in this 'compartment'), followed by activation of myosin and contraction of smooth muscle. In the peripheral vascular tree this will produce hypertension. The European Working Party on Hypertension in the Elderly (EWPHE) reported a reduction in cardiovascular mortality, and particularly in cardiac deaths, in elderly patients treated for hypertension[5]. The results were similar to the benefits reported for elderly patients in the Veterans' Administration Co-operative Group Trial[6] and the Australian Therapeutic Trial in Mild Hypertension[7]. None of these trials employed calcium antagonists and if one decides to treat an elderly hypertensive the important questions to answer are will the drug work and will it be well tolerated? Buhler[8] showed that verapamil in a dosage of 120 mg t.d.s. lowered blood pressure satisfactorily and was well tolerated by patients. He claimed that the fall in blood pressure was directly proportional to both the pre-treatment blood pressure and the age of the patient and inversely proportional to the plasma renin. Elderly hypertensives generally have low plasma renin levels. However, expressing a change in a variable against its initial value produces a 'built-in' spurious correlation due to the phenomenon of regression towards the mean[9]. Suffice it to say that calcium antagonists do lower the blood pressure in elderly hypertensives. Although there are minor pharmacokinetic differences between young and elderly patients in their handling of calcium antagonists (Table 12.3), and there

retention which results from an increase in aldosterone and can antagonize the vasoconstriction mediated partly by AII. They also improve renal perfusion.

ACE inhibitors have been used extensively in the treatment of congestive cardiac failure and have been found to be a powerful addition to the therapeutic armamentarium. The CONSENSUS trial[15] showed that the addition of enalapril to conventional drug regimes (including diuretics, digoxin and vasodilators) of patients with severe congestive cardiac failure, reduced fatality rates. This decrease in fatality was due to prevention of deterioration in cardiac failure rather than to a reduction in sudden cardiac death. Similar results had previously been shown with vasodilator therapy in the treatment of cardiac failure, but the CONSENSUS study showed enalapril to be more effective than vasodilators.

At first sight it might appear that ACE inhibitors should be used for all patients with cardiac failure. However, there is a problem in that a number of patients treated with ACE inhibitors have experienced catastrophic falls in blood pressure after the first dose[16], and in some cases this has resulted in strokes and myocardial infarction. Although one cannot predict with certainty which patients are likely to suffer such hypotensive episodes, a number of risk factors can be identified. These include high plasma renin associated with volume depletion (e.g. diuretic therapy), hyponatraemia, severe hypertension and bilateral renal artery stenosis. If possible, the risks should be reduced, for example, by reducing diuretic therapy prior to commencing treatment with an ACE inhibitor.

It has now become routine practice to admit to hospital 'at-risk' patients (mainly those in congestive cardiac failure rather than those with hypertension alone) and commence ACE inhibitor therapy with a small test dose. The present author uses 1 mg of captopril under controlled conditions with full resuscitation facilities (AII infusions, atropine, intravenous fluids and positive inotropic drugs) available.

Hypertension

The second major indication for ACE inhibitor therapy is systemic arterial hypertension. Although the elderly are typically described as having low renin hypertension, and therefore by inference low plasma AII concentrations, ACE inhibitors are as effective as diuretics in controlling hypertension in the elderly[17]. There are differences in the overall effects of ACE inhibitors in the elderly in comparison with younger patients in that the fall in blood pressure is greater and lasts longer[18]. However, if appropriately smaller doses are administered less frequently (e.g. captopril 6.25 mg b.d. or enalapril 2.5 mg daily), these differences do not prevent ACE inhibitors from being used safely in the elderly. In terms of adverse effects, the only difference between young and old is that the older patients have more episodes of mild hypotension.

The adverse effects of enalapril and captopril have now been shown to be fairly similar in frequency (Table 12.6), and the proportion of patients whose treatment has to be discontinued on account of adverse effects is similar to that seen in other forms of treatment for cardiac failure or hypertension. Fortunately the severe and potentially fatal adverse effects such as profound hypotension and angio-oedema are rare.

Table 12.6 Reported frequency of adverse reactions to angiotensin converting enzyme inhibitors

Reaction	Enalapril [19] ($n = 11\,710$) (%)	Captopril [20] ($n = 13\,295$ (%)	Captopril [21] ($n = 4124$) (%)
Rash	0.5	0.8	1.0
Angio-oedema	0.03	0.05	0.07
Hypotension	0.3	0.05	0.07
Cough	1.0	0.2	0.10
Renal function	–	0.13	0.19
Proteinuria	–	0.2	0.07
Withdrawal	4.2	7.0	2.0

Other indications for ACE inhibitors

In the future, ACE inhibitors will probably find a new therapeutic role in the treatment of chronic renal failure and diabetic nephropathy. Progressing renal failure in both these conditions is related to the remaining, normally functioning nephrons being exposed to greater pressures than normal (Figure 12.5). This increase in glomerular filtration pressure leads to glomerular hyperfiltration and eventually further deterioration in renal function. In experimental low renal mass models in rats[22] and in diabetic rats[23], treatment with ACE inhibitors has prevented deterioration in renal function as measured by urinary protein excretion. Similar results are now being seen in patients with these conditions.

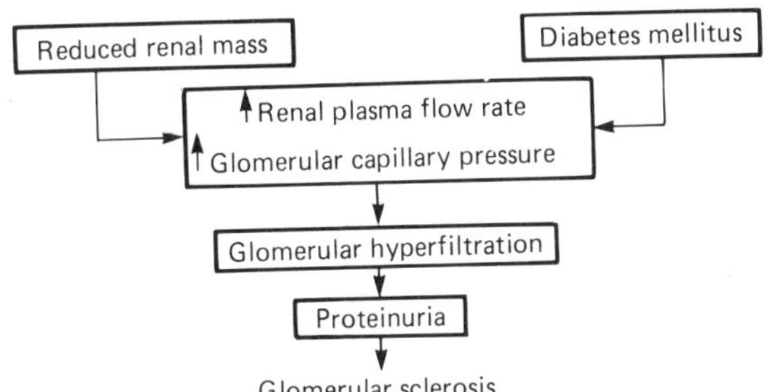

Figure 12.5 A proposed scheme for the pathophysiology of renal deterioration in reduced mass renal failure and in diabetic nephropathy

Conclusion

Clinical studies carried out among the elderly have shown that both calcium antagonists and ACE inhibitors are efficacious and well tolerated with only slight modification of dosage regimes being required. When choosing one or other of these drugs the overall clinical picture has to be appraised. For example, if the patient has angina and hypertension then a calcium antagonist is probably the better choice. If, however, the patient has cardiac failure and hypertension, then an ACE inhibitor may be better. In the case of hypertension alone either would be appropriate. One hopes that these newer drugs will not simply be added to the polypharmacy often seen among the elderly but will permit more rational and simpler prescribing.

References

1. ROSENDORF, C. In *Calcium Antagonists and Cardiovascular Disease* (ed. L. H. Opie), Raven Press, New York, pp. 323–331 (1984)
2. ANANDADAS, J. A., NARAYAN, T. R. A. and BANERJEE, A. K. *The Practitioner*, **230**, 57–60 (1986)
3. YASUE, H. In *Calcium Antagonists and Cardiovascular Disease* (ed. L. H. Opie), Raven Press, New York, pp. 117–128 (1984)
4. HUGENHOLTZ, P. G., VERDOUW, P. D., DE JONG, J. W. and SERRUYS, P. W. In *Calcium Antagonists and Cardiovascular Disease* (ed. L. H. Opie), Raven Press, New York, pp. 237–255 (1984)
5. THE EUROPEAN WORKING PARTY Mortality and morbidity results from the European Working Party on High Blood Pressure in the Elderly trial. *Lancet*, **1**, 1349–1354 (1985)
6. VETERANS' ADMINISTRATION COOPERATIVE STUDY GROUP ON ANTIHYPERTENSIVE AGENTS *Circulation*, **45**, 991–1004 (1972)
7. MANAGEMENT COMMITTEE The Australian Therapeutic Trial in Mild Hypertension. *Lancet*, **1**, 1261–1267 (1980)

8. BUHLER, F. R. Age and cardiovascular response adaptation. *Hypertension* (Suppl. 111), **5**, 94–99 (1983)
9. OLDHAM, P. D. *J. Chron. Dis.*, **15**, 969–977 (1962)
10. ABERNETHY, D. R., SCHWARTZ, J. B., TODD, E. L. *et al. Ann. Intern. Med.*, **105**, 329–336 (1986)
11. SCHWARTZ, J. B., ABERNETHY, D. R., EGAN, J. M. and MITCHELL, J. R. *Circulation*, **72** (4, Pt 2), abstract 199 (1985)
12. LEWIS, J. G. *Drugs*, **25**, 196–122 (1983)
13. SORKIN, E. M., CLISSOLD, S. P. and BROGDEN, R. N. *Drugs*, **30**, 182–274 (1985)
14. FLECKENSTEIN, A. In *Calcium Antagonists and Cardiovascular Disease* (ed. L. H. Opie), Raven Press, New York, pp. 9–28 (1984)
15. CONSENSUS. Results of the Co-operative North Scandinavian Enalapril Survival Study. *N. Engl. J. Med.*, **316**, 1429–1435 (1987)
16. CLELAND, J. G. F., DARGIE, H., McALPINE, H. *et al. Br. Med. J.*, **291**, 1309–1311 (1985)
17. WOO, J., WOO, K. S., KIN, T. and VALLANCE-OWEN, J. *Arch. Intern. Med.*, **147**, 1386–1389 (1987)
18. AJAYI, A. A., HOCKINGS, N. and REID, J. L. *Br. J. Clin. Pharmacol.*, **21**, 349–357 (1986)
19. EDWARDS, I. R., COULTER, D. M., BEASLEY, D. M. G. and MACINTOSH, D. *Br. J. Clin. Pharmacol.*, **23**, 529–536 (1987)
20. CHALMERS, D., DOMBEY, S. L. and LAWSON, D. H. *Br. J. Clin. Pharmacol.*, **24**, 343–349 (1987)
21. COOPER, W. D., SHELDON, D., BROWN, D. *et al. J. R. Coll. Gen. Pract.*, **37**, 346–349 (1987)
22. ANDERSON, S., RENNKE, H. G. and BRENNER, B. M. *J. Clin. Invest.*, **77**, 1993–2000
23. ZATZ, R., RENTZ DUNN, B., MEYER, T. W. *et al. Clin. Invest.*, **77**, 1925–1930 (1986)

Chapter 13

Ageing and receptors

Keren N. Davies and C. Mark Castleden

Introduction

There are two main reasons why drugs may have different effects in the elderly than in the young – pharmacokinetic and pharmacodynamic. The pharmacokinetic factors are those concerned with the handling of drugs, such as absorption, distribution and metabolism. Those that cause important clinical effects in the elderly have largely been identified, whilst the dynamic changes, which are the responses of the target organ to a given drug concentration, are understood only in the most preliminary way. Yet they may be far more important clinically than any kinetic changes with ageing, which can so easily be swamped by other factors, such as disease, smoking or caffeine consumption[1].

One reason for the delay in elucidating pharmacodynamic changes with ageing is the difficulty in carrying out research in this area, both *in vitro* and *in vivo*. The study of receptors, however, has recently become an accurate science and is now one way of approaching the problem. The purpose of this chapter is to discuss the achievements in this field to date, and particularly its relevance to the practice of geriatric medicine.

Definition and history

A satisfactory definition for a receptor is the particular biological macromolecule to which an agent binds with high structural selectivity and with the consequence that the characteristic biological activity of the agent is elicited. The study of radioactive-labelled ligands to receptors on cell preparations has allowed the study of receptor function to be free from altered responses caused by homeostatic mechanisms within the intact animal, but it assumes that receptors on easily accessible cells are representative of the same receptors on other locations. For example, beta-adrenoceptor function on human lymphocytes correlated with cardiac sensitivity to isoprenaline suggesting that lymphocyte beta-adrenoceptors could be studied as a representative of the beta-adrenoceptor function elsewhere in the body[2]. Binding is determined by an indirect measurement, i.e. displacement of the labelled compound from the specific saturable sites. The binding 'sites' may not necessarily be receptors, and the binding sites *in vitro* may not be available *in vivo*. Data on receptors and receptor-induced changes should therefore be regarded critically and in the context of the knowledge available about pharmaco-kinetics, pharmacodynamics and the mechanisms of actions of drugs[3].

John Langley, in 1878, advanced the theory of chemical agents inhibiting or modifying cellular response by action at specific cellular locations. By 1909 he was able to describe a receptive substance in skeletal muscle[4]. He was aware that the receptive substance had the capacity to recognize specific ligands and that the complex was able to initiate a biological response. Paul Erlich[5] introduced the term 'receptor', initially describing chemo-receptors, following his work with toxins and anti-toxins. There was then little interest in receptors following this foundation work until the 1950s.

Receptor theory and identification

Drugs, endogenous hormones and neurotransmitters act on highly selective receptors. Most receptors are thought to be localized on the surface membrane of cells[6], but some, including steroid receptors, are known to be intracellular[7]. Past theories suggested that receptors were constant in number on a cell and stationary in the cell surface membrane. If this were true, certain phenomena, including desensitization, tolerance and supersensitivity would be difficult to explain. Receptors are globular proteins embedded in a fluid lipid layer, which may be on or just below the surface membrane. Endocytosis may cause such receptors to enter cells and to be recycled or destroyed.

The sequence of events leading to a biological response after stimulation of a receptor is now known for all types of receptors, but catecholamines, ACTH and glucagon involve the adenyl cyclase system[8].

The hormone or agonist combines with the receptor inducing a change which allows coupling with a nucleotide regulatory protein. This coupled complex of hormone receptor and nucleotide is described as a ternary complex. The production of the ternary complex allows dissociation of guanine diphosphate, attached to the nucleotide protein, and its replacement by guanine triphosphate. This interaction destabilizes the ternary complex and initiates activation of adenyl cyclase, producing 3, 5 cyclic monophosphate (cAMP). Increased levels of cAMP activate protein kinases leading to phosphorylation of protein within the cell and ultimately specific response within the target tissue.

If pharmacodynamic changes are responsible for increased sensitivity to drugs with ageing, then a given concentration of drug at the receptor site must cause a greater response in an elderly person than in a younger one, assuming all other factors are constant. Unfortunately, it is extremely difficult to control for other factors. For example, Hewick and Shaw[9] showed that old rats were more sensitive to nitrazepam than younger rats and that there did not seem to be a plasma kinetic explanation. Such results mirrored previous findings in man[10]. However, the brain nitrazepam concentration in the rats was two to three times higher in the old than the young, demonstrating possible changes in the blood–brain barrier or clearance from the brain with ageing. Nevertheless, altered receptor density or affinity with ageing allows close examination of possible pharmacodynamic changes with ageing. Although researchers have identified such changes, questions still remain on how far they are important clinically or whether any such changes will be swamped by those following disease.

Interest in this field is so vast that it would be impossible to review all the progress to date. We have therefore selected some of the work on the cardiovascular and central nervous systems as examples of the progress made to date.

Cardiovascular system

Ageing reduces the response of the heart and peripheral circulation to adrenoceptor agonists and antagonists[11,12]. The increased plasma concentration of noradrenaline, both at rest and after exercise, in the elderly suggests an increased sympathetic nervous system activity[12,13]. This increased activity may lead to changes in adrenoceptors.

Beta-adrenoceptors

In 1948 Ahlquist postulated the existence of two types of adrenergic receptors, alpha and beta[14]. He distinguished them by their relative responses to a series of sympathomimetic amines.

Evidence has since emerged for there being two sub-types of beta-adrenoceptors, termed beta-1 and beta-2. Beta-receptors have been studied frequently because both the physiological, e.g. heart rate, and biological response, e.g. cAMP production, are readily measured. Specific radioligands, e.g. (3)dihydroalprenolol, are also widely available to study receptor density and affinity.

Several workers have studied cardiac beta-receptor responsiveness physiologically by measuring the dose of isoprenaline required to raise the heart rate by 25 beats per minute in man[11,12]. The first study showed a significant increase in the dose required to raise the heart rate in the elderly, implying reduced responsiveness to isoprenaline with increasing age. Birtel also demonstrated a reduction in exercise tachycardia and an increase in blood pressure response to exercise. These changes correlated with the age-related reduction in isoprenaline sensitivity. Vestal and co-workers[11] also examined the effectiveness of a given concentration of propranolol in blocking the chronotropic effect of isoprenaline, and found reduced responsiveness to propranolol with increasing age.

Interpretation of such results is not always easy because of intact compensatory mechanisms. Biological examination of beta-receptor responsiveness to isoprenaline avoids some of these difficulties. Dillon *et al.*[15] showed that lymphocytes from elderly people produced less cyclic AMP in the presence of isoprenaline than those from younger subjects. Such results could not be mirrored elsewhere when normal elderly subjects, rather than elderly patients, were used[16]. Schocken and Roth[17] initially described a reduction in beta-adrenoceptor density on lymphocytes with increasing age. This could be explained by the higher concentration of catecholamines with ageing resulting in the tissue becoming selectively desensitized to the effects of that agent. Desensitization to the stimulatory effects of beta-adrenergic agonists had been shown to be associated with a parallel fall in a number of functional beta-adrenergic binding sites. Support for this hypothesis comes from the reduction in beta-receptor binding sites seen on human lymphocyte cells when beta-agonists are given to normal people and to patients with asthma. Aarons *et al.*[18] showed that ephedrine and terbutaline, when administered for 8 days, resulted in significant decreases in the density of beta-adrenergic receptors compared to pre-treatment levels. Discontinuation of the drug resulted in the gradual return of receptor density to pre-treatment levels after about a week. Connolly and Greenacre[19] had previously shown that depression of cyclic

AMP response appeared to correlate with a degree of exposure to beta-adrenergic agonists, and confirmed that withdrawal of such drugs was followed by a reversion of the cyclic AMP response to normal values. Such results are consistent with the known response of a progressive loss of efficacy as a consequence of long-term administration of agonists acting on beta-adrenergic receptors. However, Abrass and Scarpace[20] were unable to confirm Schocken and Roth's results and found no change in receptor number or binding affinity in human lymphocytes or in the myocardium, lymphocytes or pulmonary tissue of rats with increasing age. Doyle *et al.*[21] confirmed these results in lymphocytes in man, finding that receptor density did not differ in young and elderly people. Finally, Landmann and his co-workers[22], concluded that the age-related decrease in beta-adrenergic receptor-mediated cardiovascular function did not seem to be reflected in the properties of beta-adrenergic receptors on mononuclear leucocytes.

Feldman and his colleagues[23] put forward an alternative hypothesis. Since neither receptor density nor receptor affinity for the antagonist changed with age, an alteration in beta-receptors did not involve the recognition sites of the receptor and was not due to persistent binding of endogenous agonist. Feldman suggested that reduced coupling efficiency in the beta-adrenoceptor explained the decresed sensitivity to agonists seen in the elderly, because formation of the ternary complex is a prerequisite for receptor-mediated activation of adenyl cyclase. He measured the concentration of isoprenaline required to inhibit 50% of iodohydroxybenzylpindolol binding *in vitro* on human lymphocytes, and found that the receptor affinity for agonist was correlated with age and plasma noradrenaline concentration.

In conclusion, there are major alterations in beta-adrenoceptor-agonist interactions with ageing. This does not represent an alteration in receptor density with ageing. However, it may be related at least in part to increased levels of circulating noradrenaline in down-regulation of beta-receptors.

Alpha-adrenoceptors

Since their description in 1948, alpha-receptors have also been further subclassed into alpha-1 and alpha-2, using anatomical and pharmacological material. Alpha-1 receptors are the classic post-synaptic receptors mediating smooth muscle contraction, while alpha-2 receptors have various sites, including pre-synaptic nerve terminals, where they mediate feedback inhibition of noradrenaline release. They are also found on human platelets where they mediate catecholamine-induced aggregation. Alpha-2 receptors inhibit adenyl cyclase in a variety of tissues, including platelets, whilst alpha-1 receptors appear not to interact with adenyl cyclase, but may be associated with alterations in cellular calcium fluxes.

Docherty and O'Malley[24] summed up the effect of ageing on alpha-adrenoceptors as follows; except in the eye, where there was an apparent increased responsiveness with increasing age in man, peripheral alpha-adrenoceptor responsiveness has generally been found to be either unchanged or reduced with increasing age in animals and man. It was not clear whether changes were due to alterations in alpha-receptors or whether they were due to alterations in responsiveness beyond the level of receptor. By analogy with the effect of the increased catecholamine concentrations with ageing on the beta-adrenoceptor mechanism, it is reasonable to suppose that the same increased catecholamine concentrations would reduce the response of the alpha system. Whilst there is some evidence that this is so, evidence is less convincing than with the beta-adrenoceptor system, but as with that system, the exact mechanism of any change cannot be explained on alpha-receptor density or affinity. Further studies looking at the effects of ageing on alpha-receptors are urgently required.

Central nervous system

There is a large body of evidence available suggesting that the central nervous system becomes increasingly sensitive to drugs with ageing. To date this cannot be adequately explained on pharmacokinetic grounds and it is likely that the explanation lies in pharmacodynamic changes, such as neurotransmitter levels or receptor numbers[25]. Whereas the cardiovascular system had high endogenous levels of catecholamines leading to decreased alpha- and beta-receptor response, the converse is probably true of the central nervous system, where endogenous neurotransmitters are reduced causing increased response (supersensitivity) from CNS receptors.

Dopamine receptors

There are marked changes in the nigro-striatal dopamine system which occur during physiological ageing. These include an age-dependent reduction in the number of dopamine neurones in substantia nigra, an age-dependent reduction in striatal dopamine and homovanillic acid levels, and an age-dependent decrease in the catecholamine synthesizing enzymes tyrosine hydroxylase and dopa decarboxylase in the nuclei of the striatum. The established role of diminished striatal dopamine in the pathogenesis of Parkinson's disease raises the question of whether deficiency in the normal aged brain is sufficiently great to produce clinical significant functional defects. Severe losses in dopamine can remain clinically silent, as it has been shown that just detectable symptoms of basal ganglion dysfunction, especially akinesia, are associated with a greater than 80% loss of striatal dopamine. Such losses result in a pre-synaptic overactivity in the remaining dopamine neurones indicated by a reduced ratio of dopamine to homovanillic acid, its metabolite. There is also an increase in post-synaptic dopamine receptor sites, representing a denervation supersensitivity. These two mechanisms alone may account for the inability to detect substantial striatal dopamine loss clinically. There is experimental evidence that the ageing human brain can respond normally to dopaminergic compensatory mechanisms. Whether the system would continue to work clinically well when there were increased functional requirements is unknown, as is the necessity for treatment before clinically obvious signs of Parkinson's disease develop[26].

There are several types of dopamine receptor, some of which are linked to the adenyl cyclase system and some not[27]. There appears to be a preferential loss for the post-synaptic dopamine receptor linked to adenyl cyclase. The main areas affected are the substantia nigra and the caudate nucleus[28–30]. Work in man and animals suggests that selective age-dependent decreases in transmitter receptors coupled to adenyl cyclase can occur in the absence of, or independent from, neuronal cell loss, which is seen by the retention of other biochemical markers[31].

The treatment of Parkinson's disease involves the replacement of deficient dopamine with its precursor, levodopa, or the use of a dopamine agonist, such as bromocriptine. The compensatory increase in post-synaptic dopamine receptors may explain the enhanced action of dopamine agonists in patients with Parkinson's disease, and also why lower doses may cause side-effects, such as dyskinesias.

Tardive dyskinesia

Tardive dyskinesia is another disorder of movement to which the elderly are particularly susceptible. The syndrome has been well recognized since the 1960s and often follows treatment with neuroleptics, including phenothiazines, thioxanthines and occasionally butyrophenones. The essential feature is repetitive involuntary movement choreoathetoid in type affecting the tongue, mouth, neck and extremities. The postulated pathogenesis relates to receptor changes induced by neuroleptic agents, although it is often irreversible and the chronic course would suggest a more permanent structural change.

Neuroleptic agents are central dopamine receptor blockers, and animal studies support the notion that the increased motor activity reflects supersensitivity of dopamine receptors after chronic neuroleptic treatment. Rats and mice treated chronically with neuroleptic drugs display an enhanced sensitivity to the motor stimulant effects of apomorphine, a direct dopamine receptor agonist, after neuroleptic treatment is terminated. Burt *et al.*[32] found that such treatment increased the number of dopamine receptors as measured by an increased binding of (3H) haloperidol. The change in receptor binding density was reversible. Misra *et al.*[33] studied young and old rats after treatment with fluphenazine. Both groups showed increase in dopamine-specific binding in the striatum, but the old rats also showed a substantially greater increase in adrenergic receptor binding in the cerebral cortex. Although the theory of receptor blockade, compensatory increase in dopamine receptors and supersensitivity to dopamine is attractive, it is clear that the exact nature of the cause of tardive dyskinesia, its prevalence in the elderly and its persistence after stopping neuroleptic treatment requires further study.

Benzodiazepine receptors

It is now well established that the elderly show an increased sensitivity to benzodiazepines, which has not been adequately explained on pharmacokinetic grounds[25]. In 1977 Mohler and Okada identified specific receptors in the brain for benzodiazepines[34]. These receptors are functionally linked to receptors for gamma-amino-butyric acid (GABA). GABA is a widely distributed inhibitory neurotransmitter, at 30% of synapses in the human brain[35]. It works by opening a chloride channel allowing more chloride to enter the cell, which causes hyperpolarization and decreased firing. Benzodiazepines augment this action[36]. Despite the knowledge of benzodiazepine receptors and mechanisms of action in the brain, there is little evidence for a change in either the receptors or their action with ageing. By analogy with other receptor systems, a reduction in a neurotransmitter, presumably GABA, would lead to increased sensitivity to the action of exogenous transmitters, such as benzodiazepines. To date, no such evidence exists.

References

1. JUE, S. G. and VESTAL, R. E. *Clinical Pharmacology in Drug Treatment in the Elderly* (ed. K. O'Malley), Churchill Livingstone, Edinburgh (1984), p.52
2. FRASER, J., NADEAU, J., ROBINSON, D. and WOOD, A. J. J. *J. Clin. Invest.*, **67**, 1777 (1981)
3. GARATTINI, S. and deBLASI, A. *Ageing and Drug Therapy* (ed. G. Barbagallo-Sangiorgi and A. N. Exton-Smith), Plenum Press, London (1984), p.9
4. LANGLEY, J. N. *J. Physiol.*, p. 258 (1909)
5. ERHLICH, P. *Nature*, **91**, 620 (1913)
6. ROTH, G. S. and LIVINGSTON, J. N. *Endocrinology*, **99**, 831 (1976)
7. ROTH, G. S. *Fed. Proc.*, **38**, 1910 (1979)
8. HEINSIMER, J. A. and LEFKOWITZ, R. J. *J. Am. Geriat. Soc.*, **33**, 184 (1985)
9. HEWICK, D. S. and SHAW, V. *J. Pharmacol.*, **30**, 318 (1978)
10. CASTLEDEN, C. M., GEORGE, C. F., MARCER, D. and HALLETT, C. *Br. Med. J.*, **1**, 10 (1977)
11. VESTAL, R. E., WOOD, A. J. J. and SHAND, D. G. *Clin. Pharmacol. Ther.*, **26**, 181 (1979)
12. BIRTEL, O., BUHLER, F. R., KIOWSKI, W. and LUTOLD, B. E. *Hypertension*, **2**, 130 (1980)
13. LAKE, C. R., ZIEGLER, M. G., COLEMAN, M. D. and KOPIN, I. J. *N. Engl. J. Med.*, **296**, 208 (1977)
14. ALHQUIST, R. P. *Am. J. Physiol.*, **154**, 586 (1948)
15. DILLON, N., CHUNG, S., KELLY, J. and O'MALLEY, K. *Clin. Pharmacol. Ther.*, **27**, 769 (1980)
16. KRAFT, C. A. and CASTLEDEN, C. M. *Clin. Sci.*, **60**, 587 (1981)
17. SCHOCKEN, D. D. and ROTH, G. S. *Nature*, **267**, 856 (1977)
18. AARONS, R. D., NIES, A. S., GERBER, J. G. and MOLINOFF, P. B. *J. Pharmacol. Exp. Ther.*, **224**, 1 (1983)
19. CONNOLLY, M. E. and GREENACRE, J. K. *J. Clin. Invest.*, **58**, 1307 (1976)
20. ABRASS, I. B. and SCARPACE, P. J. *J. Gerontol.*, **36**, 298 (1981)
21. DOYLE, V., O'MALLEY, K. and KELLY, J. G. *J. Cardiovasc. Pharmacol.*, **4**, 738 (1982)
22. LANDMANN, R., BITTIGER, H. and BUHLER, F. R. *Life Sci.*, **29**, 1761 (1981)
23. FELDMAN, R. D., LIMBIRD, L. E., NADEAU, J. *et al. N. Engl. J. Med.*, **310**, 815 (1984)
24. DOCHERTY, J. R. and O'MALLEY, K. *Clin. Sci.*, **68**, Suppl. 10, 133s (1985)
25. CASTLEDEN, C. M. and SWIFT, C. G. *Clinical Pharmacology in the Elderly* (ed. C. Swift), Marcel Dekker, New York (1987), p.281
26. HORNYKIEWICZ, O. *Ageing*, vol. 23: *Ageing Brain and Ergot Alkaloids* (ed. A. Agnoli), Raven Press, New York (1983), p.9
27. KEBABIAN, J. W. and CALNE, D. B. *Nature*, **277**, 93 (1979)
28. DeBLASI, A., COTECCHIA. S. and MENNINI, T. *Life Sci.*, **31**, 335 (1982)
29. MEMO, M., LUCCHI, L., SPANO, P. F. and TRABUCCHI, M. *Brain Res.*, **202**, 488 (1980)
30. MISRA, C. H., SHELAT, H. S. and SMITH, R. C. *Life Sci.*, **27**, 521 (1980)

31. SEVERSON, J. A., MARCUSSON, J., WINBLAD, B. and FINCH, C. E. *J. Neuro. Chem.,* **39**, 1623 (1982)
32. BURT, D. R., CREESE, I., SNYDER, S. H. *Science,* **196**, 326 (1977)
33. MISRA, C. H., SHELAT, H. and SMITH, R. C. *Eur. J. Pharmacol.,* **76**, 317 (1981)
34. MOHLER, H. and OKADA, T. *Science,* **198**, 849 (1977)
35. TALLMAN, J. F. and GALLAGER, D. W. *Ann. Rev. Neurosci.,* **8**, 21 (1985)
36. TALLMAN, J. F., PAUL, S. M., SKOLNICK, P. and GALLAGER, D. W. *Science,* **207**, 274 (1980)

Chapter 14

Classic genetic mutations or epimutations in ageing?
The Smith, Kline and French Lecture*

D. S. Fairweather

Is ageing genetically controlled?

There can be little doubt that inheritance plays an important part in ageing. The first line of evidence comes from the simple observation that each species has its own, 'innate' lifespan. It is true that the lifespan of many species is dependent on environmental conditions, yet maximum lifespan seems to be fixed. This is obvious in animals that live in protected environments, such as man, domestic animals and pets, and laboratory and zoo-reared species[1]. Secondly, even within one species, different, isolated, strains may have different lifespans[2]. An everyday example of this is to be found in the domestic dog. More than 100 breeds are recognized by the Kennel Club of Great Britain, and each has its characteristic lifespan, the 50% survival ranging from 6 to 12 years. This does not, of course, prove that it is really ageing that is being inherited, since it is possible that some strains die prematurely from specific diseases, as is well described in strains of laboratory mice. To establish that differences in lifespan between strains are due to differences in rates of 'intrinsic ageing' several criteria must be met (see Table 14.1). In this context perhaps the most important are: (a) that rates of accumulation of general age-related pathological change (e.g. cataract, tumours, arthritis, renal failure) are different; and (b) that the Gompertzian constants for the death rate of the two populations are different. In other words, that death results from the usual multiple causes, that the death rate in one population is at all times (after maturity) greater than in the other and that the rate-of-rise of the age-specific mortality is different in the two populations. In the case of the domestic dog the former has been established, but large numbers are required to establish the latter. In laboratory mice

*The Smith, Kline and French Lecture is an annual presentation on a topic in medical gerontology made possible by a generous donation from the Cardiovascular Forum of Smith, Kline Ltd.

171

Table 14.1 Factors necessary to establish differences in the true ageing rates of different populations

1. The mean lifespan of the populations should be different

2. The age-specific mortality curve of both populations should each be described by a Gompertz function $[M_t = M_O \times EXP(\alpha t)]$, but each with a different age-related constant (alpha)

3. Age-related physiological decrements should be similar in all respects in the two populations save that in one it is accelerated, or delayed (physiological symmetry)

4. Age-related pathological changes should be similar in all respects in the two populations save that in one it is accelerated, or delayed (pathological symmetry)

5. All members of the populations should be affected by the above processes, although to different degrees (universality of ageing)

both have been clearly established. In the case of humans, there is good evidence that family history is important in survival. Identical twins have a much closer concordance in age at death than non-identical twins; this is consistent with similar ageing rates, but does not prove genetic linkage with ageing.

The third line of evidence comes from the premature ageing syndromes in man. It is true that none of them represents acceleration of all age-related phenomena (they have been described by Martin[3] as each representing a 'segment' of overall ageing), but each has a simple pattern of inheritance suggesting that one or only a few genes are involved, although in the case of Down's syndrome it may be a whole extra chromosome. Collectively they probably fulfil criteria 3 and 4 in Table 14.1, and strongly suggest that, in humans, only a few genetic loci are important in ageing.

Since ageing, and resistance (or susceptibility) to ageing, appear to be genetic phenomena, many have argued that the nature of this resistance, and indeed of the ageing process itself, will be found by investigating genomic factors. Since ageing is a detrimental process, the obvious candidate for the cause of ageing is genomic mutation in somatic cells, and the obvious mechanism for the resistance to ageing is the ability to avoid or repair mutations. The somatic mutation theory of ageing was first formulated by Szilard[4] and later modified by him and championed by others, notably Burnet in his book *Intrinsic Mutagenesis, a Genetic Approach to Aging*[5]. Hart and others[6–9] provided apparently confirmatory evidence by showing that there is a good correlation between the ability to repair DNA and lifespan. Thus it came about that the obvious mechanism seemed confirmed and became firmly established in people's minds, so that now some even talk about 'ageing mutations' (meaning probably irreparable mutations). The logic of this is compelling: ageing is a genetic phenomenon, DNA must get irreparably damaged in time, DNA repair is related to ageing, therefore ageing is due to DNA damage, and thus mutations – but it is quite wrong.

Difficulties with the somatic mutation theory of ageing

If ageing is primarily due to somatic mutations then the following criteria should be satisfied:

1. Cellular death will be related to the number of indispensable genes (for each species), to whether they are duplicated (i.e. autosomal or X-linked) and to the mutation rate. Given the number of relevant genes and their disposition, an estimate may be made of the required mutation rate for a given mean lifespan: this should accord with experimental observation.
2. The greater the 'spare genetic capacity' (for example, diploid versus haploid or polyploid versus diploid), the greater should be the lifespan.
3. Similarly, lifespan should be related to the inherited fault load. Presumably mutations are most significant when both alleles are mutant (i.e. the individual is homozygous for a fault). Thus the higher the initial load of heterozygous faults, the shorter should be the lifespan.
4. It is crucial that lifespan should be related to the ability to avoid or repair mutations.
5. It is also crucial that mutations should be shown to occur or accumulate in relation to other ageing changes.
6. Promotion of mutation should shorten lifespan due to accelerated ageing.

There are other, more formal attributes of an ageing process which are given in Table 14.2, but the above are of particular relevance to mutations, and over the past 20 years each of these postulates has been investigated, with surprising results. Szilard recognized in his original publication[4] that the then known mutation rate was improbably low to account for ageing on any reasonable assumptions. He therefore postulated that each 'ageing mutation' would have to be a 'hit' damaging a number of genes at a time, for example a whole section of a chromosome. Holliday has used the

Table 14.2 Attributes of an ageing process

1. The process must be shown to occur with age

2. The process must be shown to be able to cause the normal age-related decrements (qualitative equivalence)

3. Decrements quantitatively similar to those occurring during normal ageing must be shown to be produced by the equivalent degree of the process as has been found to occur during ageing (quantitative equivalence)

4. Acceleration of the process should accelerate all facets of ageing

5. Retardation of the process should delay all facets of ageing

6. Natural variations in ageing should be associated with similar variations in the process concerned

in vitro ageing model of Hayflick[10] to test the somatic mutation theory. He found that to account for the known *in vitro* lifespan of human fibroblasts one has to postulate either an impossibly high number of indispensable genes (10^5), or a mutation rate of between 10^{-3} and 10^{-4}, which is a thousand times the known mutation rate. It seems unlikely that the mutation rate is the same for all genes. The possibility exists that there are a few important genes with mutation rates that are very much higher than those that have been measured, but this is also unlikely. However, Holliday and Kirkwood[11] also found that calculations (based on the rate of accumulation of mutations) predicted that early during *in vitro* culture a significant proportion of cells should be non-viable, and experiments do not confirm this.

Similar *in vitro* ageing experiments have been done with cells made polyploid, for example by cell fusion[12,13]. Contrary to prediction, none of these studies showed that lifespan was longer in the polyploid cells. Such experiments with intact animals are not generally possible, but there does exist a haploid variant of the wasp *Habrobracon*. The haploid male is more sensitive to the mutagenic effect of ionizing radiation, just as one would predict from the lack of duplicated genetic information available, but its lifespan is just the same as that of the diploid varieties, whether irradiated or not[14].

An alternative to proposing a very high number of indispensable genes, or a very high mutation rate, is to assume a high rate of inherited heterozygous faults. In humans, the general rate of genetic disorders does not suggest that this is the case, but a detailed examination of inherited fault loads is difficult. In experimental animals a classic way of investigating this is to look at the effect of inbreeding. Inbred strains may, initially, have a high level of inherited fatal faults, but repeated inbreeding will tend to reduce these, and in any event, inbred adults will have a low frequency of heterozygous faults which are potentially fatal (simply because they have survived to adulthood and with inbreeding faults are likely to be homozygous or non-existent, and not heterozygous). Two differing inbred strains will have a different pattern of inherited faults, but the adults of both will have a lower rate than outbred, or wildtype adults. The somatic mutation theory predicts that inbred adults should have a longer lifespan than outbred adults, and that hybrids of two outbred strains will have an intermediate survival. In fact, in both insects and mammals exactly the opposite is the case. This is not at all easy to reconcile with the somatic mutation theory[15].

Much has been made of the pioneering work of Hart *et al.* on DNA repair processes and ageing. They used ultraviolet light to induce DNA damage and measured the incorporation of 3H-thymidine into DNA, to assess overall repair[6]. They found a good correlation between the logarithm of 'maximum lifespan' and relative DNA repair for seven mammalian species from the short-lived shrew to man. There are now, however, important reasons to doubt the significance of this. First, ultraviolet light mainly produces a very specific lesion in DNA (pyrimidine dimers) which can either be directly reversed by a specific enzyme system, or be incorporated in a patch of excision repair (in which case new thymidine will be incorporated and measured by the 3H-thymidine uptake assay). Most somatic cells are never exposed to ultraviolet light, even the dividing cells of the optic lens are in the periphery and protected by the iris, and it is hard to think that this type of challenge is typical of that occurring throughout life in the majority of somatic cells. More recently, Vijg and colleagues have re-examined the repair of ultraviolet-induced DNA lesions in the rat and found that although rat cells are somewhat slower at repair than human ones, their viability following exposure to ultraviolet light is exactly the same as human cells, and given long enough their repair is just as good[16]. Further, rat cells exposed to ultraviolet light *in vivo* (as opposed to irradiation *in vitro*) have much more active repair than cultured cells, indicating that some of the previously reported effects may be artefactual[16]. There are undoubtedly some differences in DNA repair between rodents and man but the relationship between repair and ageing is not good[17] and anyway it may be a secondary effect of ageing (see below).

What about mutations occurring *in vivo*? In cultured cells, mutations do appear to accumulate in the last 20% or so of lifespan, and although it is possible that this might be the cause of cells' finally ceasing to divide, the kinetics of mutation accumulation in cultured cells are quite wrong (see above) and it is possible that the observed mutations are the result of ageing changes in the cells, perhaps propagated through errors in synthetic pathways. There is some evidence for accumulation of mutation in the X-chromosome gene HPRT in the circulating lymphocytes of ageing humans[18] but it is also possible that the observed changes (which are too small for mutation to be a primary determinant of ageing) are the result of a change in the circulating pool of cells that is being sampled, and that these changes are due to a yet more fundamental ageing change. In experimental animals, convincing evidence for age-related accumulation of mutations is lacking[19].

For almost every physiological or metabolic 'repair' process there is an associated theory of ageing. Accelerating death by accelerating a putative ageing process is a prerequisite for establishing the importance of the process concerned. However, such an experiment does not prove that in practice the process is responsible for what we see as ageing. It is also necessary to show that the process occurs at an appropriate rate *in vivo* and that normal modulators of the process modulate ageing (see Table 14.2). Ionizing radiations and mutagenic drugs in appropriate doses can certainly shorten lifespan but whether they accelerate ageing is quite another matter. In insects, low dose radiation actually lengthens lifespan, and as indicated above, in the haploid wasp there is no association between the mutagenic effect of ionizing radiation and lifespan. In rodents, radiation has been shown to reduce lifespan and possibly to accelerate ageing, but this remains controversial, and such an effect may not be due to the induction of classic mutations (see below).

It can thus be seen that not one prediction of the somatic mutation theory of ageing has been clearly substantiated. Some may hang on to the theory by citing methodological problems with each of the points raised above, yet when all the evidence seems contradictory it is surely sensible to look elsewhere. Even if we admit that somatic mutations could bring about ageing changes, that somatic mutations do occur, and even that their accumulation accelerates in old age, this is not the same as admitting that these mutations are the cause of ageing because the rate of accumulation may be far too low. Methuselah at 969 years may have aged because of mutation, but whether we do so at three score and ten is another matter.

Epigenetic information and epimutations

It has long been known that DNA contains some modified bases, but it is only recently that the importance of base modification has become clear. In vertebrate DNA there are some very rare base modifications present, but it is not known if these play any functional role. By far the most abundant modified base is 5-methylcytosine; about 5% of all cytosines are methylated. Cytosines are only methylated in 5'CpG3' couplets and symmetrically on both DNA strands as shown in Figure 14.1. More than 50% of such couplets are methylated. Even so, it may be that only a few methylation sites are functionally important. It appears that certain methylation sites in the 5'-flanking regions of some genes exert control on gene expression such that methylation is associated with repression (a silent gene) and demethylation with expression (an actively transcribed gene)[20]. Methylation may be responsible for the tissue-specific activation of genes that occurs during normal development, and ageing might represent corruption of this controlling mechanism.

The information provided by the methylation pattern has come to be known as the 'epigenetic code', and alterations to it as 'epimutations' to distinguish them from classic mutations. A classic mutation involves the alteration of the sequence of bases in DNA, but an epimutation does not affect this code because 5-methylcytosine behaves (codes) in exactly the same way as cytosine during transcription (i.e. it is transcribed into guanine of RNA). It is important to understand how cytosine comes to be modified by the action of the maintenance methylase enzyme, and this is illustrated in Figure 14.1 (Pathway A). The maintenance methylase enzyme will only efficiently methylate DNA if it is already hemimethylated (i.e. has an asymmetric methyl group on one strand). Another enzyme exists in some cells which can insert a methyl group in totally non-methylated DNA; this is referred to as *de novo* methylation.

The fact that cytosine becomes methylated after semiconservative synthesis rather than being incorporated directly is significant. There is a short delay in methylating the nascent strand after DNA synthesis, and this provides a method for recognizing which of the strands is new, and thus helps in excision repair of mismatched bases or segments (see Figure 14.2). But perhaps most important of all, it also provides an important difference in the inheritance of epigenetic information.

There is now a body of information which suggests that epigenetic information may be relevant to ageing. Wilson and

Jones[21] showed that 5-methylcytosine levels fell during *in vitro* ageing of fibroblasts of human and rodent origin. Fairweather *et al.*[22] demonstrated the same for another human fibroblast cell strain, and also that this is related to cell division and not only to time in culture. The mechanism for this and its relation to the Hayflick limit is illustrated in Figure 14.1, Pathway B. The same cells transformed and immortalized by infection with SV-40 virus have stable methylation over many hundreds of cell divisions[23]. Likewise, transformed Syrian hamster fibroblasts have stable

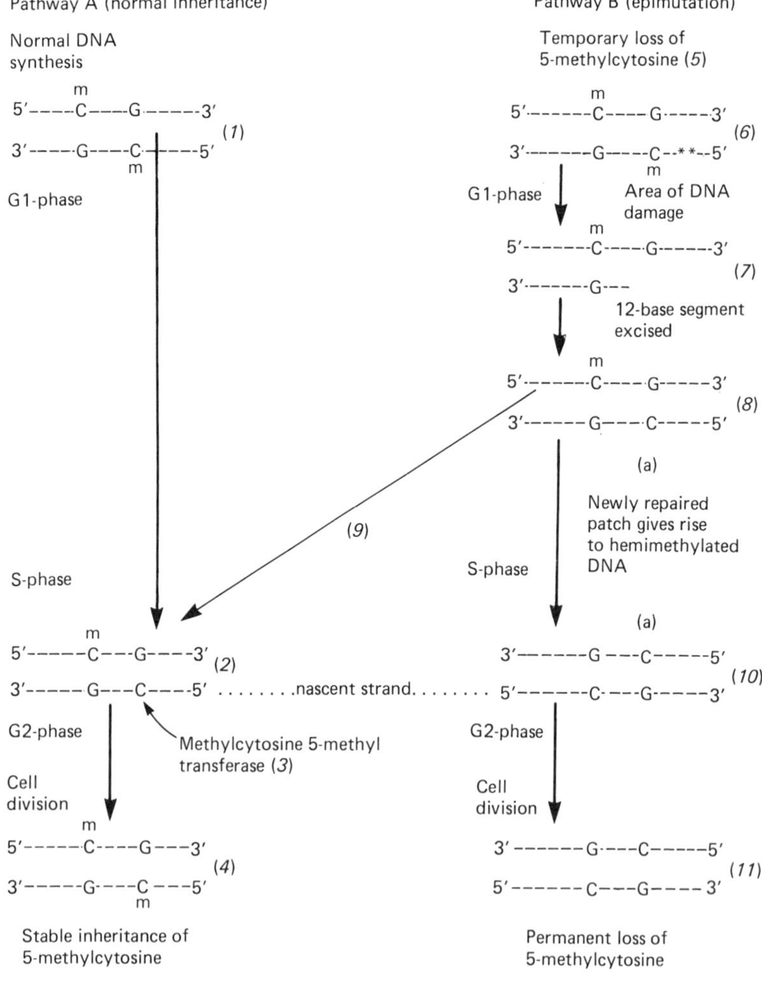

methylation, as do cells derived from the same cell strain which are immortal but not fully transformed. NIH 3T3 cells[21] also have stable methylation. This suggests that stable methylation is a feature of the immortality and not just an associated feature of transformation.

Methylation has not yet been studied in detail during *in vivo* ageing but preliminary data from a study by Catania and Fairweather (in preparation) suggest that there are changes in some tissues. *In vitro* measurements show that the age-related decline in methylation brings the level close to that which has been found fatal for cells, and this may well explain death at the Hayflick limit[22,24].

The rate of loss of methylation has been measured in mouse, hamster and human cells. In each case the rate of loss was related to the *in vitro* lifespan of the cells concerned, which is consistent with postulate 6 in Table 14.2. Postulate 4 (acceleration of ageing by acceleration of the process) has been investigated by the use of the artificial demethylating agent 5-azacytidine, and this drug has

Figure 14.1 *(opposite)* Inheritance of epigenetic information and epimutations. (*1*) In vertebrates, 5-methylcytosine occurs exclusively in 5′CpG3′ doublets, and symmetrically on both DNA strands. (*2*) Normal, semiconservative DNA synthesis with incorporation of 2′-deoxycytidine into the nascent strand (to pair with guanine in the old strand) in place of 5-methyl-deoxycytidine that had been present in the old complementary strand. (*3*) The maintenance cytosine 5-methyl transferase enzyme (Cyt5MT) attaches a methyl group on the 5 position of cytosine to match symmetrically the methylation pattern of the old strand. (*4*))Faithful inheritance of the mother-molecule's methylation pattern. (*5*) Loss of 5mC from one strand leads to hemimethylated DNA (*8*). This loss of 5mC might be due to: (i) inefficiency of Cyt5MT enzyme; (ii) single strand breaks (which appear to inhibit this enzyme; (iii) the spontaneous deamination of 5-methylcytosine to thymine giving rise to the mismatched pair G-T, which is not correctable and; (iv) the base being included in a segment of excision-repair shortly before S-phase (which is illustrated here). (*6* and *7)* Many forms of DNA damage (e.g. a thymidine dimer (*6*)) distort the helix, and may be repaired by excision of a 12-base segment either side of the lesion(*7*). (*8*) The repaired patch will initially have cytosine inserted in place of 5-methylcytosine (i.e. be hemimethylated, see (*2*) and (*3*)). If this process occurs sufficiently close to S-phase that the maintenance methylase does not have time to act, then the two strands will provide different templates for semiconservative synthesis. (*9*) The methylated strand provides an accurate substrate for semiconservative DNA synthesis as above (*2*), and preservation of the methylation pattern (*3* and *4*). (*10*) The demethylated ('repaired') strand provides an apparently normal substrate for semiconservative DNA synthesis, but the methylation pattern is not re-established because the Cyt5MT will effectively only act on hemimethylated DNA and the methyl group at site (*a*) is absent. (*11*) Half the daughters from this cell will be permanently demethylated at this site. It is therefore S-phase, and cell division, which perpetuates what would otherwise be a temporary loss of 5-methylcytosine. This fits with the Hayflick limit which is also dependent on cell division

Original DNA strand and methylation pattern

```
                m
(1)    5'T  – A – C – G – T – A – C – G3'
       3'A  – T – G – C – A – T – G – C5'
                                m
```

Inaccurate DNA synthesis during S-phase with mispaired bases (*)

```
                m
(2)    T  – A – C – G – T – A – C – G
       G  – C – G – C – A – T – G – C
       *      *
```

Nascent DNA strand is recognized by repair enzymes because of its lack of methylation

```
                m
(3)    T  – A – C – G – T – A – C – G
       ..................................  A – T – G – C
       Excised portion
```

```
                m
(4)    T  – A – C – G – T – A – C – G
       A  – T – G – C – A – T – G – C
       Resynthesis
```

```
                m
(5)    T  – A – C – G – T – A – C – G
       A  – T – G – C – A – T – G – C
                                m
       Remethylation
```

Figure 14.2 Methylation-directed DNA repair. A, adenine; C, cytosine; G, guanine; T, thymine; m, methylated cytosine (5-methylcytosine); * misincorporated bases. (1) Cytosine is only methylated in 5'CpG3' couplets, and the pattern is symmetrical on both strands. (2) Although DNA polymerase probably has its own proofreading function, some mispaired bases are incorporated (*). These may distort the helix, or be otherwise recognized, but either strand could be at fault. In order to correct the mispairing the strand which is in error must be identified. Lack of methylation on the new strand might be the marker which directs the enzyme(s) to the erroneous strand[29]. (3) A short segment of the new DNA may be excised and (4) a new attempt at correct synthesis made. (5) Finally the new strand becomes fully methylated

been found to produce a striking reduction in the *in vitro* lifespan of human fibroblasts[22,25] which is related to the degree of hypomethylation induced[22]. Such a striking effect on lifespan following a single treatment with a drug has not been observed before.

It has not proved possible to retard this process, so that postulate 5 (Table 14.2) cannot be investigated. The commitment theory of ageing[26] suggests that fibroblast cultures consist of a mixture of a few 'uncommitted cells' which have high proliferation potential and may be analogous to 'stem cells', and a great preponderance of 'committed', ultimately mortal cells. The nature of commitment might be the loss of *de novo* methylating activity, since immortal cells must presumably have such activity in order to keep their methylation levels stable. It is interesting that the recently described rat cell system which has reversible immortality[27] might provide the answer to this: the acquisition of immortality may be associated with acquisition of *de novo* methylating activity, and the reversion to mortality with the loss of it.

Some paradoxes explained

The loss of epigenetic information in 5-methylcytosine thus fulfils many of the requirements of a basic ageing process (Table 14.2). It can also explain several of the apparent paradoxes demonstrated by the data on somatic mutations.

The rate and kinetics of 'mutations'

Classic mutations are essentially all-or-nothing. That is, the mutation consists of, at the very minimum, a change in a base-pair which either gives rise to a structural error in the protein, or alters gene expression or regulation. A mutation in a silent part of DNA is irrelevant for our purposes. It is known, however, that epigenetic switches may not be like this. The relevant methylation sites are mainly in the 5' flanking region of a gene, and more than one site may have to be methylated (or demethylated) to affect expression. Thus, loss of one or more methylated sites may have no immediate phenotypic effect, but renders the cells more liable to such phenotypic change in the future when the final methylated site is lost (see Figure 14.3). Such a process is analogous to the multistep process of carcinogenesis, and produces exponential phenotypic effects from a process that is essentially linear. Calculation from the data of methylation loss shows that the epimutation rate is about 10^{-3}, which is a thousandfold the somatic mutation rate. It is certainly sufficiently frequent to explain age-related changes, and the multistep process illustrated above can explain the high viability of cells during middle lifespan in culture, whereas somatic mutations cannot.

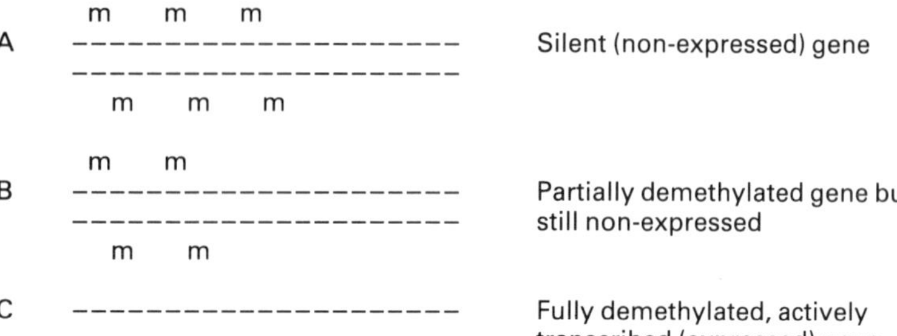

Figure 14.3 DNA methylation and gene expression

Inherited 'fault load'

It should be possible to investigate inherited fault load, but unfortunately only a small proportion of methylation sites are functionally important, so although several cell types exist with very different methylation levels, it does not follow that in all of these cells the important methylation sites are differently methylated.

It is possible, however, that epimutation may be able to explain the great paradox of the differences in lifespan between inbred and outbred strains, and at the same time point to a basic mechanism for 'resetting the ageing clock' during meiosis and reproduction.

It is known that recombination during meiosis is far from random, and only involves coding regions of DNA. Holliday[28] has proposed that crossing-over is controlled by specific sites for each gene which may be identical with, or associated with, the 5′ controlling regions of genes. Recombination involves the formation of a segment of hybrid DNA in which the coding sequence for each crossing pair is provided from one gene only (as is obviously the case) whereas the controlling region may have one strand contributed from each crossing pair. Such a mechanism provides an obvious solution to the problem of site-specific recombination and is shown diagrammatically in Figure 14.4. The epigenetic information on the controlling region from one gene will thus provide the pattern necessary to repair that lost from the corresponding region of the other gene and *vice versa* (Figure 14.4). During the development of germ cells it would be unlikely that random loss of methylation would be present at identical sites in two alleles and therefore this proposed 'meiosis-associated repair process' could be very efficient.

Genes with normal methylation pattern

Gene A

```
m   m   m
r r r r r r r r r r c c c c c c c c c c c c c c c c c c c c c
r r r r r r r r r r c c c c c c c c c c c c c c c c c c c c c
  m   m   m
```

Gene B

```
m   m   m
RRRRRRRRRRCCCCCCCCCCCCCCCCCCCCCC
RRRRRRRRRRCCCCCCCCCCCCCCCCCCCCCC
  m   m   m
```

Genes after germ-line development and ageing showing random demethylation

```
      m
r r r r r r r r r r c c c c c c c c c c c c c c c c c c c c c
r r r r r r r r r r c c c c c c c c c c c c c c c c c c c c c
      m
```

```
  m   m
RRRRRRRRRRCCCCCCCCCCCCCCCCCCCCCC
RRRRRRRRRRCCCCCCCCCCCCCCCCCCCCCC
    m   m
```

Genes after crossing over

Gene B crossed with A (1)

```
      m
r r r r r r r r r r CCCCCCCCCCCCCCCCCCCC
RRRRRRRRRRCCCCCCCCCCCCCCCCCCCCCCCC
  m   m
```

Gene A crossed with B (1)

```
  m   m
RRRRRRRRRRc c c c c c c c c c c c c c c c c c c c
r r r r r r r r r r c c c c c c c c c c c c c c c c c c c c
      m
```

Methylation pattern after the action of maintenance methylase (2)

```
m   m   m
r r r r r r r r r r CCCCCCCCCCCCCCCCCCCC
RRRRRRRRRRCCCCCCCCCCCCCCCCCCCCCCCC
  m   m   m
```

```
m   m   m
RRRRRRRRRRc c c c c c c c c c c c c c c c c c c c
r r r r r r r r r r c c c c c c c c c c c c c c c c c c c c
  m   m   m
```

Figure 14.4 Repair of epigenetic defects by recombination during meiosis. R,r, sequences in the 'recombinator' site; C,c, sequences in the gene coding regions; m, methylated cytosine in a CpG couplet. (1) One strand of the recombinator sequence is contributed by gene A (r) and the other by gene B (R), while the coding sequences derive from *either* by gene A (c) *or* gene B (C). (2) The epigenetic pattern can be re-established by using information from the recombinator site of one allele to repair the defects in the other

This immediately provides an explanation for the effect of inbreeding on lifespan. Inbred strains will tend to be 'homozygous' for epigenetic defects (as well as classic genetic defects), and thus meiosis-associated repair will not be possible, and inbred individuals will start with a high rate of epigenetic defects and therefore have a shortened lifespan. Different inbred strains will have different epigenetic faults, and therefore crosses between two inbred strains will have a longer lifespan than the two parent strains. However, outbred animals, or the wild type, will have the lowest number and most heterozygous epigenetic faults, and so will have a longer lifespan than either the inbred strains or their hybrids. This is in accord with experimental observation and the possibility that inbred strains may have different levels of methylation at crucial sites is potentially testable.

Meiosis-associated repair of epigenetic defects cannot, however, explain the persistence of methylated cytosines in coding regions, and also in highly reiterated (or nonsense) DNA sequences. Since this has persisted during evolution despite the propensity for 5-methylcytosine to be lost (by deamination to thymine), there must be a specific mechanism to effect this, and consequently some advantage in the persistence of these methyl groups. Possible advantages are alterations to the physical structure of DNA which 5-methylcytosine imparts, or its ability to affect its interaction with protein. An alternative is that methylation of cytosine can provide information to direct correction of errors induced by DNA synthesis, as do methylated adenines in prokaryotes. This process is illustrated in Figure 14.2 above. Evidence that methylated DNA is better repaired than non-methylated DNA has been reported[29], but it is possible that there are other, as yet undiscovered advantages of methylation which could account for this persistence.

DNA repair may also be important in the loss of 5-methylcytosine. The carbon–carbon bond in 5-methylcytosine is too stable thermodynamically to cleave spontaneously even under *in vivo* conditions, so that some other mechanism may be responsible for the age-related decline that has been observed. Spontaneous deamination of 5-methylcytosine to thymine undoubtedly occurs (possibly 1% over a human lifespan) but at an insufficient rate to account for the rate of loss observed in dividing cells. Several DNA lesions are repaired by excision of a short segment of one strand (up to 12 bases long)[23]. If such a process occurs shortly before S-phase, and a methylated cytosine is included in the patch, then the maintenance methylase may not have sufficient time to act before semiconservative DNA synthesis fixes the methylation loss in one of the new strands. Thus DNA damage may, secondarily, lead to loss of methylation, and strand-breaks in particular reduce the efficiency of the maintenance methylase enzyme. Since a major action of X-rays on DNA is to induce strand breaks, it is possible that some of the lifespan-shortening effect of ionizing radiation is related to hypomethylation.

Conclusion

There can be no doubt that mutation in somatic cells occurs during ageing, and that the vast majority of mutations will be detrimental. However, the rate at which errors will be introduced by mutation is orders of magnitude lower than the error-rate of the translational process itself[23], and the kinetics of mutation do not fit with experimental observations. In addition, none of the predictions of the somatic mutation theory of ageing has been borne out by experimental data. If ageing is fundamentally an energy-saving strategy, as implied by Kirkwood[30], then failure of genomic maintenance (and thus mutation) may simply be a byproduct of ageing: there is no need for good maintenance in a species that dies or ages for other reasons. Nevertheless, mutation may play a role, particularly in very old age.

Table 14.3 Summary of important differences between genetic and epigenetic information

1. Although epigenetic information is dependent on coding bases (in this case on the presence of 5'CpG3' pairs) it is essentially independent of the coding sequence

2. Methylation occurs as a separate step after DNA synthesis, and processes ensuring the integrity of the genetic code are different from those maintaining the epigenetic code

3. Genetic mutation and epimutation may occur as separate processes

4. DNA repair (that is genomic maintenance) may actually bring about epimutation because of the necessary delay between repair and remethylation

5. The inheritance of genetic and epigenetic information may be different

6. Meiosis may enable the epigenetic pattern to be restored

7. Epigenetic switches may require several groups to be altered for exerting their maximal phenotypic effects, thus producing a multistage, delayed alteration to gene expression

By contrast to somatic genetic mutations, epimutations can provide a solution to some of the anomalies of the previous theory. Furthermore, they may be interlinked with the most basic processes of meiosis, crossing-over and sexual reproduction; these factors are summarized in Table 14.3. The mechanism whereby meiosis and sexual reproduction 'resets the ageing clock' has been an enigma to gerontologists. We now have a testable theory to work on: the next few years may provide the answer.

References

1. COMFORT, A. *The Biology of Senescence*, 3rd edn, Churchill Livingstone, London (1979)
2. BELLAMY, D. In *Principles and Practice of Geriatric Medicine* (ed. M. S. J. Pathy), Wiley, London, pp. 67–104 (1985)

3. MARTIN, G. M. In *Genetic Effects on Aging* (ed. D. Bergsma and D. E. Harrison), A. R. Liss, New York, pp. 5–39 (1978)
4. SZILARD, L. *Proc. Natl Acad. Sci.*, **45**, 30–45 (1959)
5. BURNET, M. *Intrinsic Mutagenesis: a Genetic Approach to Ageing*, MTP Press, Lancaster (1974)
6. HART, R. W. and SETLOW, R. B. *Proc. Natl Acad. Sci.*, **71**, 2169–2173 (1974)
7. HART, R. W., SACHER, G. A. and HOSKINS, T. L. *J. Gerontol.*, **34**, 808–817
8. HART, R. W., D'AMBROSIO, S. M., NG, K. J. and MODAK, S. P. *Mech. Ageing Devel.*, **9**, 203–223 (1979)
9. HART, R. W. and MODAK, S. P. *Adv. Exp. Med. Biol.*, **129**, 123–137 (1980)
10. HAYFLICK, L. *Cell Res.*, **37**, 614–636 (1965)
11. HOLLIDAY. R. and KIRKWOOD, T. B. L. *J. Theor. Biol.*, **93**, 627–642 (1981)
12. THOMPSON, K. V. A. and HOLLIDAY, R. *Exp. Cell Res.*, **112**, 281–287 (1978)
13. HOEN, H., GRYANT, E. M., JOHNSTON, P. *et al. Nature*, **258**, 608–609 (1975)
14. CLARKE, A. M. and RUBIN, M. A. *Rad. Res.*, **15**, 244–253 (1961)
15. MAYNARD-SMITH, J. *Proc. R. Soc. (Lond.)*, **157**, 115–127 (1962)
16. VIJG, J. and KNOOK, D. L. *J. Am. Geriat. Soc.*, **35**, 532–541 (1987)
17. KATO, H., HARDA, M., TSUCHIYA, K. and MORIWAKA, K. *Jap. J. Genet.*, **55**, 99–108 (1980)
18. EVANS, H. J. and VIJAYALAXMI *Nature*, **292**, 601–605 (1981)
19. HORN, P. L., TURKER, M. S., OGBURN, C. E. *et al. J. Cell. Physiol.*, **121**, 309–315 (1984)
20. BIRD, A. *Nature*, **307**, 503–504 (1984)
21. WILSON, V. L. and JONES, P. A. *Science*, **220**, 1055–1057 (1983)
22. FAIRWEATHER, D. S., FOX, M. and MARGISON, G. P. *Exp. Cell Res.*, **168**, 153–159 (1987)
23. FAIRWEATHER, D. S. and EVANS, J. G. In *The Metabolic and Molecular Basis of Acquired Disease* (ed. R. D. Cohen, K. G. M. M. Alberti, B. Lewis and A. M. Denman), Baillière Tindall, London (1988)
24. FLATAU, E., GONZALES, F. A., MICHALOWSKY, L. A. and JONES, P. A. *Mol. Cell. Biol.*, **4**, 2098–2102 (1984)
25. HOLLIDAY, R. *Exp. Cell Res.*, **166**, 543–552 (1986)
26. KIRKWOOD, T. B. L. and HOLLIDAY, R. *J. Theor. Biol.*, **53**, 481–496 (1975)
27. AMTMANN, E., MULLER, K., KNAPP, A. and SAUER, G. *Exp. Cell Res.*, **161**, 541–550 (1985)
28. HOLLIDAY, R. *Science*, **238**, 163–170 (1987)
29. HARE, J. T. and TAYLOR, J. H. *Proc. Natl Acad. Sci.*, **82**, 7350–7354 (1985)
30. KIRKWOOD, T. B. L. In *Advanced Geriatric Medicine 5* (ed. R. C. Tallis and F. I. Caird), Churchill Livingstone, London, pp. 109–116 (1986)

Index